MW00619149

Choosing a Natural Immunomodulator
A Scientific Approach

Vaclav Vetvicka

Author's Disclaimer

This book is not intended as medical advice. It is written solely for informational and educational purposes. Please consult a health professional before taking any natural modulator. Because there is always some risk involved, the author and publisher are not responsible for any adverse effects or consequences resulting from the use of any of the suggestions or preparations described in this publication. Neither the publisher nor author advocate the use of any particular product, but believe the information presented in this book is important enough that it should made available to the public.

Choosing a Natural Immunomodulator

A Scientific Approach

Printed in the United States of America

Cover: Kalima by Rayonier

Interior: 70# Spring Forge Offset by Pixelle

Font: Georgia

Library of Congress Control Number: 2019904984

ISBN: 978-0-9841445-3-2

TABLE OF CONTENTS

1

PREFACE

In the current digital age, everybody has heard something about natural immunomodulators, but the real knowledge is limited and confusing. Some people do not believe at all, while some have unrealistic expectations. There is a lot of information on the web, but some of the information is too scientific, and therefore difficult for the general public to understand, and some of the information is commercially-driven and more often than not inaccurate. With more than 30 years of supplements research under my belt, I am confident that I can provide both scientific and reliable information about natural supplements to the general public. Provided with my information, readers can decide whether or not to supplement their food with any of these substances.

During my 30 years of supplement studies, I collaborated with numerous companies around the world, including the Laboratoires Goémar in Saint-Malo, where I studied the effects of marine glucans with Dr. Jean-Claude Yvin and Dr. Edouard Panak. Subsequently, I was also involved with the Brazilian glucan manufacturer Biorigin and French Groupe Roullier in Saint-Malo, doing additional research on using glucan and/or flavoids in combination with other bioactive materials that might increase their already impressive biological actions. In additional collaborations, I evaluated the biological properties of natural immunomodulators made and sold in the United States, Brazil, Turkey, Croatia, Germany, Taiwan, South Korea, Japan and the Czech Republic.

All these collaborations were entirely science-driven. I am not selling glucan (or any other supplement) and I never have, nor am I endorsing any particular brand. I wrote this book objectively and completely without any profit motive. Therefore, all information is for educational purposes only. Any commercial name used in this book is mentioned only as a result of my own extensive testing.

After reading this book, one should have enough information to clearly and confidently decide if any particular supplement is worth the effort. The second question this book answers is: for whom is the book intended? It is for students who have an interest in, or are required to learn about nutritional supplements; for nutritionists, looking for an improved nutritional regime; for readers seeking new ways to improve their health and to understand the confusing field of natural immunomodulators; and for physicians who are interested in supplements and their action, but have no time to immerse themselves into the vast universe of scientific publications.

Readers will easily notice that individual chapters differ in their size, with the chapter on glucan being the longest. The explanation is simple – first of all, I did most of my research in the field of natural supplements on the biological and immunological effects of glucan. And second – glucan is the most studied natural immunomodulator, with more than 40,000 studies published in peer-reviewed scientific journals. In addition, glucan is one of the only natural supplements which has no possible negative side effects and has appropriate scientific protocols for research and marketing.

A dietary supplement is a manufactured product intended to supplement the diet when taken by mouth. The class of nutrient compounds includes vitamins, minerals, fiber, fatty acids and amino acids. Dietary supplements can also contain substances that have not been confirmed as being essential to life, but are marketed as having a beneficial biological effect, such as plant pigments or polyphenols. Animals can also be a source for supplement ingredients. Supplements can be sold individually or in combinations of different nutrients. In the United States and Canada, dietary supplements are considered a subset of food, and are regulated accordingly. Currently, there are more than 50,000 dietary supplement products marketed just in the United States alone and over 50% of the American population takes at least one dietary supplement each day. My hope is to help the general public find substances that have consistent and beneficial characteristics and activities.

This book was written primarily to give the reader a complex overview of the most important natural immunomodulators and supplements, their activities, potentials and possible setbacks. I am keeping the text simple, but giving full details, including full scientific references, so the readers can judge the evidence for themselves. This literature is far from comprehensive, but represents carefully chosen, most relevant studies.

2

INTRODUCTION

To use natural products as a possible remedy is weaved into the history of mankind. People have been appealing to nature for curing various diseases since ancient times. The first documented history of plant preparation and medicinal use is a record on Sumerian clay tablets from the period of 4000 B.C. A written Indian document talking about medicinal effects of mushrooms is app. 5000 years old. Indian Ayuveda and traditional Chinese Medicine can serve as an example of healing trends which have been developed through empirical experience. A physician of Marcus Aurelius emphatically pioneered the treatment of diseases by using the specific diets Galen of Pergamum. Several centuries later, J. Lind used 200-year-old Dutch knowledge using the benefits of citrus fruits to the health of the sailors on long voyages, and conducted one of the first large-scale clinical medical trials. Japanese legend indicates that monkeys without cancer or any other disease fed on mushroom *Lentinula edodes*. Medicinal plants are commonly used for the therapy of various diseases and represent significant part of old folk remedies. The continuous development of medicine and science was associated with the development of synthetic medicinal products, and plant therapy was slowly pushed aside. Alternative therapy, also known as complementary medicine, refers to a variety of therapies and practices that usually falls out of the scope of traditional medicine. These health practices include acupuncture, homeopathy, herbal medicine, special diets, and aromatherapy, and are frequently used both in addition to and in place of, conventional treatment. Dietary supplements are preparations that conceptually fall into an in-between category that lies somewhere between food and drugs. Quite often, the line is not distinct. Hundreds and hundreds of different botanicals are used in complementary and alternative medicine or as a part of healthy nutrition. While there's some anecdotal evidence and an increasing number of interested researchers and lately even more clinical studies of the mechanisms on how different herbs elicit clinical effects, they are not well described and remain largely unknown.

Out of an estimated 250,000 flowering plant species globally, between 50,000 and 70,000 are known to be used in traditional and modern medicine. That does not mean they are all active, as only about 6% have been screened for biological activity. Despite this lack of knowledge, botanical supplements are used worldwide with the expectation of boosting immune responses and reducing various pathogen-associated symptoms. This is particularly true in third world nations, where the World Health Organization estimates suggest that up to 80% of population relies on herbs for primary health care needs. In the United States, the prevalence of herbal remedy use increased by 380% between 1900 and 1997 (Eisenberg et al., 1998). In Europe, over 2 billion dollars are spent on herbal products and in Germany alone, approximately 10% of the pharmaceutical market is herbal-based medicine. In the United States, it is estimated that up to one third of the entire population used complementary and alternative medicine in the last 12 months. Many products are rushed on the market and heavily marketed, without significant studies backing the claims. Commercially it works, as the sales of pomegranate-based supplements raised from $84,000 in 2001 to $66 million in 2005 in United States alone.

The use of herbal supplements in the United States is steadily growing by approximately 20% per year. There are more than 50,000 dietary supplement products marketed just in the United States, where about 50% of the American adult population consumes dietary supplements. In the United States, the Dietary Supplement Health and Education Act of 1994 (DSHEA) provides this description: "DSHEA defines the term "dietary supplement" to mean a product (other than tobacco) intended to supplement the diet that bears or contains one or more of the following dietary ingredients: a vitamin, a mineral, an herb or other botanical, an amino acid, a dietary substance for use by man to supplement the diet by increasing the total dietary intake, or a concentrate, metabolite, constituent, extract, or combination of any of the aforementioned ingredients. Furthermore, a dietary supplement must be labeled as a dietary supplement and be intended for ingestion and must not be represented for use as conventional food or as a sole item of a meal or of the diet. In addition, a dietary supplement cannot be approved or authorized for investigation as a new drug, antibiotic, or biologic, unless it was marketed as a food or a dietary supplement before such approval or authorization. Under DSHEA, dietary supplements are deemed to be food, except for purposes of the drug definition." It is therefore important to remember that herbals are classified as food supplements and not considered medicine, they are not regulated by FDA and are subject to much looser requirements. It is important to note that during preparation of this law, more letters were written in favor of nutritional supplements than were written to protest the Vietnam War (Soller, 2000).

Unlike the situation in the United States, herbal medicine is heavily regulated in Germany. Commission E, working since 1978, is part of the Federal Health Agency and controls the scientific studies on each herb. There must be an absolute proof of safety and reasonable certainty of efficacy, or the access to the market is blocked.

Scientific research supports the biological activity of many of food phytochemicals, but the health claims attributed to the final marketed supplements have often little or even doubtful scientific foundation. This reality is mostly due to the fact that a lot of the evidence is derived from pure chemicals used in animal studies, whereas clinical trials are scarce.

Our book could not focus on all possible herbs and natural molecules with possible biological activities and used on current markets. Among plants and herbs which we overlooked but are still worth mentioning are *Glycyrrhiza glabra* (licorice or sweetwoods) with potential anti-inflammatory and hepatoprotective effects; *Withania somnifera* (Ashwagandha) with potential anti-inflammatory, diuretic and anti-cancerous effects; *Azadirachta indica* with possible effects on ulcers and malaria; *Zinziber officinale* (ginger) with effects on the gastrointestinal tract, rheumatism and inflammation; garlic with some anti-helminth and immunomodulatory properties; *Nigella sativa* (Black cumin) with the ability to inhibit bacterial infections; *Aloe vera* used in wound healing and treatment of skin infections; and *Hydrastic canadensis* (Goldenseal) containing alkaloids with antibacterial properties (for recent review see Tiwari et al., 2018). Another subject of considerable interest is cocoa, a product consumed since 600 BC. It has considerable antioxidant properties and possesses strong regulatory activities by influencing the production of inflammatory cytokines by macrophages and other cells. The action is most probably attributed to the content of flavonoids (Ramiro-Puig and Castel 2009). Honey is another immunomodulator known and used for centuries by probably all cultures for treatment of various disorders including wounds and burns. It offers a broad spectrum of anti-microbial properties and promotes faster wound healing.

In addition to the anti-microbial effects, honey has multifactorial immunomodulatory properties including regulation of production of important cytokines. One of the less known, but still important, immunomodulators is leptin. Leptin is an adipocyte-derived hormone that links nutritional status with neuro-endocrine and immune functions. It regulates energy homeostasis. Originally described as an anti-obesity hormone, it has been subsequently shown to influence also basal metabolism, hematopoiesis, thermogenesis, reproduction, and angiogenesis.

However, even with widespread use and acceptance, and despite research efforts, a complete understanding of the biochemistry and mechanisms of action regarding most herbal remedies has remained largely unknown. Due to low or nonexistent standardization, you may never know what is in the capsule. When LA Times analyzed 10 different brands of St. John's Wort by mass spectrophotometry, results showed that the potency ranged from 20 % to 140% of the claimed potency (Brody, 1999).

Reports of contaminants such as pesticides, heavy metals, and bacteria are common. Another problem might be the real concentration in the commercial product. It is always beneficial to be sure that the manufactures can provide a Certificate of Analysis and that the Good Manufacturing Practices are observed. In addition, there are reports of the presence of lipopolysaccharide in medicinally prepared extracts of some plants and herbs (Denzler et a., 2010), most probably not as a result of contamination during harvesting and preparation, but due to the symbiotic endophytic bacteria present in the plants. While the amount of LPS found might not be dangerous when consumed orally, it might be responsible for some biological effects observed in animal studies. Similarly, some products labeled as ginseng contain mandrake, which is scopolamine or snake root (reserpine). In both cases the reason is simple – the source is cheaper than real ginseng. Additional impurities in herbs include narcotics, antibiotics, steroids and non-steroidal anti-inflammatory drugs (Sigel 1978, Capobianco et al., 1993).

The population growth in the developing world and the increasing interest in the industrial nations have greatly expanded the interest in natural remedies. At least 20% of adults in the United States have taken a dietary supplement in the past six months and over 4 billion dollars is spent annually on herbal supplements alone.

There is intense public debate over the efficacy and safety of herbal and dietary supplements and over the absence of requirements for rigorous testing of the efficacy, content, and/or safety of these compounds. However, they are classified by the FDA as food, therefore, they are not subjected to the same evaluation as drugs. To be removed from the market, supplements must be proven unsafe and the proof submitted to the Secretary of Health and Human Services.

For patients taking prescription drugs, if little or no data is available on the potential herb-medication interaction, the conservative approach is to recommend against supplement use. In addition, product quality is important. An estimated 16 million adults combine supplements with prescription medicines. At the same time, the amount of studies suggesting modulation of drug effects by herbal remedies is increasing. Herbs with the potential to significantly modulate the activity of drug-metabolizing enzymes and/or the drug transporters include ginkgo, garlic, *Echinacea*, ginseng, St. John's wort, and kava (Spareboom et al., 2004).

Another often raised question is the use of herbal (or any other) supplements during pregnancy or during lactation. The first part is easy, we clearly do not know enough to be sure that the supplements will not harm the fetus, so none of the supplements are recommended for pregnant women. In lactation, the possible danger is smaller. However, the study evaluating the safety of popular herbal supplements in lactating women reached the conclusion that not enough information is available and more research is necessary before any guidance could be given (Amer et al., 2015). There have been concerns about the purity of various herbs, particularly found in foreign markets, with contamination by heavy metals (Winslow and Kroll, 1998). Another problem is that most herbals are manufactured by small companies without the resources and/or know-how to sponsor and perform large-scale studies, both experimental and clinical. In addition, it is usually difficult to patent natural molecules, strongly lowering potential interest of pharmacological companies.

Clearly, some herbs are medically useful (for review see Espin et al., 2017, Tiwari et al., 2018). However, even with demonstrated effects, the potential negative effects might overcome the usefulness of them, therefore caution is advised. Many patients use dietary supplements in conjunction with traditional pharmaceuticals often for the same health conditions. Drug interactions can and probably will occur. It is extremely important to check for any new symptoms when using herbs, vitamins, or dietary supplements.

There is already solid scientific basis to support biological activity of some natural food supplements, but the task is far from completed. Clearly, the public would benefit from increased regulation, forcing manufacturers to ensure that herbs contain pure ingredients. More and better designed clinical trials need to be carried out with particular emphasis on the bioavailability and metabolism. Importantly, the public should avoid following various web doctors with doubtful qualifications.

References

Amer, M.R., Cipriano, G.C., Venci, J.V., Gandhi, M.A.: Safety of popular herbal supplement in lactating women. J. Hum. Lact., 31: 348-353, 2015.

Brody, J.E.: American gamble on herbs as medicine. New York Times 9: 2, 1999.

Capobianco, D.J., Brizis, P.W., Fox, T.O.: Proximal muscle weakness induced by herbs. N. Engl. J. Med., 329: 1430, 1993.

Denzler, K.L., Waters, R., Jacobs, B.L., Rochon, Y., Langland, J.O.: Regulation of inflammatory gene expression in PBMCs by immunostimulatory botanicals. Plos One, 5, e12561, 2010.

Eisenberg, D.M., Davis, R.B., Ettner, S.I., Appel, S., Wilkey, S., Van Rompay, M., Kessler, R.C.: Trends in alternative medicine use in the United States, 1990-1997: result of follow-up national survey. JAMA, 28: 1569-1575, 1998.

Espin, J.C., Garcia-Conesa, M.T., Tomas-Barberan, F.A.: Nutraceuticals: Facts and fiction. Phytochemistry, 68: 2986-3008, 2017.

Ramiro-Puig, E., Castell, M.: Cocoa: antioxidant and immunomodulator. Br. J. Nutr., 101: 931-940, 2009, doi:10.1017/S0007114508169896.

Siegel, R.: Kola, ginseng, and mislabeled herbs. JAMA, 237: 24-25, 1978.

Soller, R.W.: Regulation in the herb market. The myth of the "unregulated" industry. HerbalGram, 49: 64-67, 2000.

Spareboom, A., Cox, M.C., Acharya M.R., Figgs, W.D.: Herbal remedies in the United States: Potential adverse interactions with anticancer agents. J. Clin. Oncol., 22: 2489-2503, 2004.

Towari, R., Latheef, S.K., Ahmed, I., Iqbal, A.M.N., Bule, M.H., Dhama, K., Samad, H.A., Karthik, K., Aagawany, M., El-Hack, M.E.A., Yatoo, M.I., Farag, R.: Herbal immunomodulators – A remedial panacea for designing and developing effective drugs and medicines: Current scenarios and future prospects. Curr. Drug Metabl., 19: 264-301, 2018.

Winslow, L.C., Kroll, D.J.: Herbs as medicines. Arch. Intern. Med., 158: 2192-2199, 1998.

3

ASTRAGALUS

Astragalus propinquus (better known as *Astragalus membranaceus)*, is widely distributed throughout the temperate region of the world. Its dried root was first documented in Shennong Bencao Jing (published ~200–300 CE). *Astragalus,* commonly known as Mongolian milkvetch (Figure 1), or as Huang Qi in traditional Chinese medicine, is one of the oldest and most frequently used botanicals for Asian medicine in China, Korea, Japan, and other Asian countries. The root is the most commonly used part.

The bioactive constituents in the root are complicated. The root contains more than 100 chemical compounds including polysaccharides, flavonoids, astragalosides, amino acids, and trace elements. Scientific investigations during the last two decades have revealed much insight into the pharmacological fractions, with most of the attention focused on polysaccharides, as their concentration is higher than all the other bioactive components combined (Tian et al., 2012). The results of these studies support the idea that the most important bioactive components are probably the numerous polysaccharides. Four distinct polysaccharides were isolated and characterized from a water extraction of *Astragalus* roots. Ethanol precipitation resulted with four polysaccharides differing in molecular weight, monosaccharide composition, and immunobiological activities.

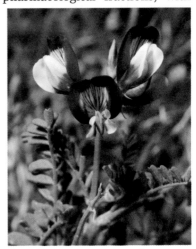

Figure 1 *Astragalus* (Milkvetch)

Besides polysaccharides, saponins represent another molecule with suggested biological effects. Some studies found that these saponins inhibit experimentally-induced inflammation (Wang et al., 2016). The downside of these experiments lies in fact that they measure only *in vitro* effects on the increase in inflammation, and not the possible effects *in vivo*. An interesting approach used *Astragalus* as part of the delivery vehicle for a vaccine. Studies conducted on chickens showed a potentiation of antibody response against avian influenza virus, H5N1, by oral supplementation (Abdullahi et al., 2016).

To add to the confusion, some authors believe that astragaloside is responsible for the biological effects (Qi et al., 2017). So, either *Astragalus* has several distinct types of bioactive molecules, all able to affect the same reactions, or there are errors in the preparation and purification processes. In addition, the effects of purified components are always better than effects of crude *Astragalus* extract alone. That is hard to explain, as a combination of three molecules with the same effects should be stronger than the individual parts.

Among many reported bioactivities of *Astragalus*, the most prominent are anti-oxidant, anti-viral, anti-hypertensive, anti-inflammatory, anti-diabetic, anti-tumor, and immunomodulatory activities. A summary of the biological activities of the polysaccharides revealed that these activities fully corresponded to the activities found in *Astragalus* extracts (Jin et al., 2014). The study, however, found no relation between structure and function, as every manuscript evaluated and described different compositions of tested polysaccharides.

Most of the research regarding the effects of *Astragalus* has been focused on its antitumor effects. The results are often contradictory. Some studies suggested that these effects are mediated via stimulation of T lymphocytes, while others showed activation of B lymphocytes but no activation of T lymphocytes at all.

Despite the fact that inhibition of cancer growth belongs among demonstrated action of *Astragalus*-derived polysaccharides, the pharmacological effects are less clear. One of the polysaccharides was used in treatment of hepatocellular carcinoma in mice. The most effective dose was 400 mg/kg. In addition to inhibition of tumor growth, the study also found strong stimulation of immunity including cytokine production (Lai et al., 2017). In cancer studies, results showed robust stimulation of immunity leading to inhibition of angiogenesis of tumors (Zhang et al., 2018). If confirmed, it might suggest a novel use for *Astragalus* extracts.

Astragalus has been widely used in veterinary clinics, and shown to enhance the immune response to several vaccines against viruses including Newcastle disease, foot-and-mouth disease, and avian influenza. A detailed study showed that *Astragalus*-derived polysaccharide enhanced the immune response to avian bronchitis virus vaccinations in chicken (Zhang et al., 2017).

Several studies have focused on colitis, reporting that the extract manifested both preventive and therapeutic potential in experimentally-induced colitis, most probably via anti-oxidation and modulation of colonic cytokines. A more detailed study showed that these effects were mediated by promotion of T helper cell transcription factors and by potentiating a shift toward T helper 2 phenotype. If confirmed, it would be a step towards using this polysaccharide in treatment of colitis (Gao et al., 2016).

One of the few studies that focused on elucidation of mechanisms of action showed that *Astragalus* polysaccharides exert their immunomodulatory effects via TLR4-mediated MyD88-dependent signaling pathway (Zhou et al., 2017). Despite a solid experimental design and a high quality of research, this study also suggested potential involvement of other pathways, as some of the results were confusing and some even contradictory.

Understanding which molecule is responsible for the described effects could strongly increase the interest of pharmacological companies and the potential for a drug development from *Astragalus*. In addition, precise dosing of *Astragalus* in humans remains unclear, because it is mainly used in multiherb preparations and clinical trials are scarce. In mice, the LD50 dose is greater than 15 g/kg, strongly suggesting that *Astragalus* is safe.

In conclusion, *Astragalus* is safe, but the lack of knowledge of the active ingredients, mechanism of action, and which reactions are really affected, significantly lower the enthusiasm for this food supplement.

References

Abdullahi, A.Y., Kallon, S., Yu, X., Zhang, Y., Li, G.: Vaccination with *Astragalus* and ginseng polysaccharides improves immune response of chicken against H5N1 Avian influenza virus. BioMed Res. Int., 2016, doi:10.1155/2-16/`510264.

Gao, Y.J., Zhu, F., Gian, J.M., Dai, J.Y.: Therapeutic and immunoregulatory effect of GATA-binding protein-3/T-box expressed in TA-cell ratio of *Astragalus* polysaccharides on 2,4,6-trinitrobenzene sulfonic acid-induced colitis in rats. Chin. J. Integr. Med., 12: 918-924, 2016.

Jin, M., Zhao, K., Huang, Q., Shang, P.: Structural features and biological activities of the polysaccharides from *Astragalus membranaceus*. Int. J. Biol. Macromol., 64: 257-266, 2014.

Lai, X., Xia, W., Wei, J., Ding, X.: Therapeutic effect of *Astragalus* polysaccharides on hepatocellular carcinoma H22-bearing mice. Dose-response: Int. J., 15: 2017, doi:10.1177/1559325816685182.

Qi, Y., Gao, F., Hou, L., Wan, C.: Anti-inflammatory and immunostimulatory activities of astragalosides. Am. J. Chin. Med., 45: 1157-1167, 2017.

Tian, Q.E., Li, H.D., Yan, M., Cai, H.L., Tan, Q.Y., Zhang, W.Y.: *Astragalus* polysaccharides can regulate cytokine and P-glycoprotein expression in H22 tumor-bearing mice. World J. Gastroenterol., 18: 7079-7986, 2012.

Wang, Y., Ren, T., Zheng, L., Chen, H., Ko, J.K., Auyeung, K.K.: *Astragalus* saponins inhibits lipopolysaccharide-induced inflammation in mouse macrophages. Am. J. Chin. Med., 44: 579-593, 2016.

Zhang, P., Wang, J., Wang, W., Liu, X., Liu, H., Li, X.: *Astragalus* polysaccharides enhance the immune response to avian infectious bronchitis virus vaccination in chickens. Microbiol. Pathogen., 111: 81-85, 2017.

Zhang, X.P., Li, Y.D., Luo, L.L., Liu, Y.Q., Li, Y., Guo, C., Li, Z.D., Xie, X.R., Song, H.X., Yang, L.P., Sun, S.B., An, F.Y.: *Astragalus* saponins and liposome constiture an efficacious adjuvant formulation for cancer vaccines. Cancer Biotherap. Radiopharmaceut., 33: 25-31, 2018.

Zhou, L., Liu, Z., Wang, X., Yu, S., Long, T., Zhou, X., Bao, Y.: *Astragalus* polysaccharides exerts immunomodulatory effects *via* TLR4-mediated MyD88-dependent signaling pathway *in vitro* and *in vivo*. Scientific Rep., 7, 2017, doi:10.1038/srep44822.

4

CAT'S CLAW

Two species of Cat's Claw, *Uncaria guianesis* and *U. tomentosa* (Figure 2 and 3) have been used for medicinal purposes by Peruvian Indians for over 2000 years, and it gained a name: "life-giving vine of Peru." It is a woody vine that derives its name from hook-like thorns that grow along the vine and resemble the claws of a cat. The vine contains a clear watery sap; it grows wild in the upper Amazon region of Peru and neighboring countries, and can reach several inches in diameter and 1,000 feet in height. Today, these plants are attracting attention in the West because of their potential immunostimulant properties. The attention started when Keplineger began studying its properties in 1974. In some European countries (e.g., Austria and Germany), Cat's Claw can be dispensed only with a prescription. A boiled decoction or extract is produced from the inner bark of the vine, and is used for medicinal purposes. Lately, extracts from roots have gained popularity, too. Some researchers suggest that these plants can enhance immune reactions due to the content of various flavonoids, sterols, carboxyl alkyl esters, triterpene, and/or alkaloids found in the stalk bark and roots. Some studies have found 17 different molecules, while others have found 29 molecules, still others found over 50 components. The most investigated of the active constituents for immunomodulating activities are pentacyclic oxindole alkaloids.

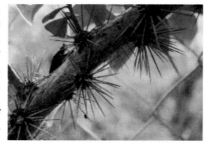

Figure 2 Cat's Claw
Uncaria guianesis

19

Lately, it was found that two chemotypes of *U. tomentosa* with different alkaloid patterns occur in nature. The roots of one type contain pentacyclic oxindoles, the other contains tetracyclic oxindole. Recent studies have shown that the tetracyclic alkaloids exert antagonistic effects on the action of the peptacyclic ones, making clear that mixtures of these two types of drugs are unsuitable for medicinal uses (Reinhard, 1997).

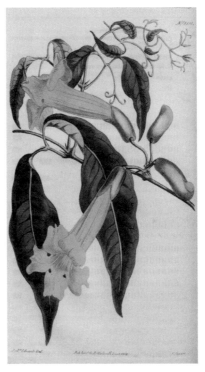

Figure 3 Cat's Claw *U. tomentosa*

Some of the more recent studies focused on water-soluble extracts, which contain no measurable levels of alkaloids, but still have biological functions. Subsequent studies revealed that the responsible molecule is quinic acid esters. Results showing inhibition of cell growth without causing cell death offer an interesting possibility for DNA repair (Sheng et al., 2005).

The pharmacological actions of Cat's Claw include anti-oxidant properties, anti-inflammatory activity, cytoprotection, immunomodulation, and anti-hypertensive effects. Some studies found stimulation of phagocytosis (Groom et al., 2007) and suppression of TNF-α leading to anti-inflammatory effects; for review, see Williams et al. (2001). The anti-oxidant properties, however, were confirmed only *in vitro*. Regarding the anti-oxidant effect, oxidative stress is a unifying feature of all cardiovascular risk factors and a factor that is elevated in response to neurohormonal abnormalities in heart failure; it is important to remember that despite the recent years of progress, the successful use of oxidative stress markers is still far away. So in this regard, the major question remains—if it is true (as so many studies confirm) that oxidative stress is critical in the development of cardiovascular problems, why do so many anti-oxidant trials fail? The answer is probably that, in this particular regard, the anti-oxidants work fine *in vitro*, but reactive oxygen species (ROS) responsible for oxidative stress are produced continually, so anti-oxidants also have to be present continually and in relatively high concentration to be able to reduce possible spikes in ROS levels. Loading cells with too much anti-oxidant might block too much of the ROS and prevent them from their essential biochemical pathways.

Using a fish model, scientists observed increased growth and stimulated immune activity in fish when challenged with a bacterial infection (Yunis-Agionaga et al., 2015); whereas, limited studies suggested possible direct anti-microbial activity.

Cell culture experiments showed that the hot water extract inhibited cell division and NF-kB activity without inducing cell death. These effects might explain some of the previously reported anti-inflammatory actions. Direct comparison of two extracts and two pure alkaloid preparations on peripheral mononuclear cells found that all four agents modulated immunobiochemical pathways induced by interferon (Winkler et al., 2004). The results suggested that these effects might be beneficial in some autoimmune diseases, infections, and coronary heart disease. In addition, it seems that there is no need for isolation of active substances.

Some studies suggest possible anti-apoptotic functions, which might lead to DNA repair in chemotherapy-damaged cells. Detailed studies confirmed treatment with Cat's Claw increased apoptosis and sensitized cells to radiation-induced cell death (Allen et al., 2017). These results were further supported by a study comparing different ways to isolate the extract. The study found the traditional methanol extract is the least active. The other extracts clearly demonstrated induction of apoptosis and explained the effects are manifested both via receptor-mediated pathways and mitochondria-mediated pathways.

This makes it the first real elucidation of possible mechanisms of action (Cheng et al., 2007). The problem with these studies is that they were all *in vitro* only, so we do not know if oral supplementation will have comparable results. In addition, these studies often lack negative controls or at least other types of cell lines. The study comparing effects of water extracts on squamous carcinoma cells found clear stimulation of apoptosis and resulting inhibition of proliferation, but at the same time, found similar, albeit lower, effects on normal skin cell line (Ciani et al., 2018). This puts significant doubts on possible development of this extract into a clinically useful drug. Only one study showed that orally administered extracts improved proliferation of myeloid progenitor cells and increased neutrophil numbers in mice with experimentally-induced neutropenia (Farias et al., 2011).

A systematic review of possible interactions with anti-retroviral treatment showed that Cat's Claw significantly increased the levels of anti-retrovirals in patients (Jalloh et al., 2017), suggesting that these patients should be carefully monitored for possible adverse effects. Another negative effect was found in patients suffering from Parkinson disease, where oral intake of Cat's Claw resulted in worsening of motor symptoms (Cosentino and Torres, 2008). Evaluations of safety and clinical efficiency are still insufficient to draw firm conclusions. In addition, the experimental results are often dependent upon the nature of the preparation use; i.e., tablets, extracts, decoction. Because of the lack of adequate clinical trials, more studies are needed to establish a place in therapy.

In summary, the health promoting effects of Cat's Claw are still not fully established. Similarly, we do not know which molecule is responsible for the attacks. The possibility of negative side effects suggests the need for caution.

References

Allen, L., Buckner, A., Buckner, E.A., Cano, P., Lafrenie, R.M.: *Uncaria tomentosa* (Willd. ex Schult.) DC (*Rubiaceae*) sensitizes THP-1 cells to radiation-induced cell death. Pharmacognosy. Res., 9: 221-229, 2017.

Cheng, A.C., Jian, C.B., Huang, Y.T., Lai, C.S., Hsu, P.C., Pan, M.H.: Induction of apoptosis by *Uncaria tomentosa* through reactive oxygen production, cytochrome c release, and caspases activation in human leukemia cells. Food Chem. Toxicol., 45: 2206-2218, 2007.

Ciani, F., tafuri, S., ATroiano, A., Cimmino, A., Cimmino, A., Fioretto, B.S., Guarino, A.M., Pollice, A., Vivo, M, Evidente, A., Carotenuto, D., Calabro, V.: Anti-proliferative and anti-apoptotic effects of *Uncaria tomentosa* aqueous extract in squamous carcinoma cells. J. Ethnopharmacol., 211: 285-294, 2018.

Cosentino, C., Torres, L.: Reversible worsening of Parkinson disease motor symptoms after oral intake of *Uncaria tomentosa* (cat's claw). Clin. Neuropharmacol., 31: 293-294, 2008.

Farias, I., do Carmo Araujo, M., Zimmermann, E.S., Dalmora, S.L., Benedetti, A.L., Alvarez-Silva, M., Asbahr, A.C.C., Bertol, G., Farias, J., Schetinger, M.R.C.: *Uncaria tomentosa* stimulates the proliferation of myeloid progenitor cells. J. Ethnopharmacol., 137: 856-863, 2011.

Groom, S.N., Johns, T., Oldfield, P.R.: The potency of immunomodulatory herbs may be primarily dependent upon macrophage activation. J. Med. Food, 10: 73-79, 2007.

Jalloh, M.A., Gregory, P.J., Hein, D., Cochrane, Z.R., Rodriguez, A.: Dietary supplement interactions with antiretrovirals: a systematic review. Int. J. STD AIDS, 28: 4-15, 2017.

Reinhard, K.H.: *Uncaria tomentosa* (Willd.) D.C.: Cat's claw, Una de Gato, or Saventaro. J. Altern. Compl. Med., 5: 143-151, 1999.

Sheng, Y., Akesson, C., Holmgren, K., Berngelsson, C., Giamapa, V., Pero, R.W.: An active ingredient in Cat's Claw water extracts. Identification and efficacy of quinic acid. J. Ethnopharmacol., 96: 577-584, 2005.

Williams, J.E.: Review of antiviral and immunomodulating properties of plants of the Peruvian rainforest with a particular emphasis on Una de Gato and Sangre de Grado. Alternative Med. Rev., 6: 567-579, 2001.

Winkler, C., Wirleitner, B., Schroecknadel, K., Schennach, H., Mur, E., Fuchs, D.: *In vitro* effects of two extracts and two pure alkaloid preparations of *Uncaria tomentosa* on peripheral blood mononuclear cells. Planta Med., 70: 205-210, 2004.

Yunis-Aguinaga, J., Claudiano, G.S., Marcusso, P.F., Manrique, W.G., de Moraes, J.R.E., de Moraes, F.R., Fernandes, J.B.K.: *Uncaria tomentosa* increases growth and immune activity in *Oreochromis niloticus* challenged with *Streptococcus agalactiae*. Fish Shelfish Immunol., 47: 630-638, 2015.

5

CHLORELLA

Microalgal food supplements are becoming increasingly popular due to their promising biological effects and high nutritional value. *Chlorella* is a single-cell green freshwater algae. They are eukaryotic unicellular animals that have been documented to exist at least one billion years ago. The cells are spherical and non-motile with sizes ranging from 2–8 mm. It has a very hard outer shell, making it almost completely indigestible to humans, so supplements have to undergo a special process cracking the shell for enhanced digestibility. Figure 4 *Chlorella*

Chlorella (Figure 4) represents a high-energy source as it contains essential amino acids, proteins, and carbohydrates. It is also a good source of various vitamins (such as B1, B2, B3, B6, B9, C, D, E, and H), chlorophyll, carotene, ascorbic acid, lutein zeaxanthin, iron, and magnesium. Due to the high nutritional content, *Chlorella* is sometimes marketed as a "natural all-in-one supplement." Besides general benefits in nutrition, some immunoenhancing effects have been reported. A clinical study found increased natural killer (NK) cell activity and elevated production of cytokines such as IFN-γ, IL-12 and

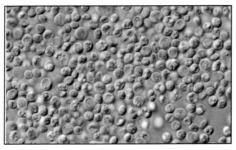

Figure 4 *Chlorella*

IL-17. Interestingly, de Souze Queiroz et al. (2013) found that *Chlorella* supplementation reduced the depression of myelopoiesis caused by stress.

Like with most natural materials, the individual product can significantly vary depending on cultivation, harvesting, and processing. Some studies have revealed that the contents of commercial products can consist of 7–88% proteins or of 6–38% carbohydrates, making the claims about biological activities highly questionable. This is based partly on the different isolation techniques and partly on the legendary adaptability of this species. This fact makes any serious evaluation of possible biological effects difficult. First, it is generally difficult to explain function without understanding the mechanisms of action and, second, we do not know how different batches differ in their content, even from the same manufacturer.

In a fish model, *Chlorella* supplementation resulted in amelioration of arsenic-induced immunosuppression and oxidative stress. However, to achieve these results, *Chlorella* had to reach 10% of fish diet.

As the immunostimulating effects of *Chlorella* are still questionable, some animal experiments have reported small increases of physical stamina, suggesting more nutritional use of these algae. Similarly, a finding of improvements of immune function in protein-deficient mice (An et al., 2010) is more in line with improving nutritional deficiencies, which commonly result in immunosuppression. There exists a possibility that the clinical trial participants had inadequate nutritional status and the nutrients in the *Chlorella*-derived supplement attenuated their health problem. All these findings support using *Chlorella* as more of a functional food than an immunostimulant. A small human study found that daily supplementation with a high dose of 30 tablets increased the production of salivary IgA (Otsuki ety al., 2011). Necessitating the use of heavy doses further supports possible nutritional effects, as with other highly active substances, the immune system needs only a few milligrams.

There is documentation that supplementation with *Chlorella* results in reduction of blood sugar levels, improvements of animal growth, increased hemoglobin concentration, and lower cholesterol levels; for review, see Kay (1991). Overall, the studies evaluating the effects on dyslipidemia are confusing, as some studies reported decreased cholesterol or triglyceride levels and some studies found little or no effects (Panahi et al., 2016). When taken together with statins, the effects seem to be higher, without increasing possible negative side-effects of statins. The effects are highly dose-dependent, suggesting that the positive effects are caused by a high volume of fiber present in *Chlorella* supplements.

Interestingly, Bae et al. (2013) reported inhibitory effects on allergic immune response via inhibition of serum IgE overproduction, offering a completely different window into potential use of *Chlorella*. Possible mechanisms might involve inhibition of histamine release from mast cells involved in allergic reaction. Oral supplementation also suppressed experimentally-induced atopic dermatitis-like conditions in mice. The mechanisms of action included reduction of eosinophil and mast cell infiltration into the skin and downregulation of several important chemokines (Kang et al., 2015), further supporting the use in allergies. With respect to the immune system, the results are confusing and most probably dose dependent. Whereas, low concentration can support the immune system, higher concentrations will suppress it. A randomized, double-blinded, placebo-controlled trial found beneficial immunostimulatory effects of short-term supplementation (Kwak et al., 2012), mostly as activation of the NK cell functions and early inflammatory response. In a report of Ehrlich ascites tumor-bearing animals, feeding with *Chlorella* extract resulted in prolonged survival (Justo et al., 2001). A different species, *Chlorella sorokiniana*, decreased cancer cell viability *in vitro* and slowed the growth of lung cancer *in vivo* (Lin et al. 2017). An older study showed strong improvements in survival for Ehrlich ascites tumor, mouse leukemia, and mouse mammary carcinoma (Miyazawa et al., 1988) after only five injections or five days of oral supplementation. If true, *Chlorella* really could be a wonder drug against cancer. However, these results were never repeated. In addition, the authors used either whole cells or a heat-extracted substance with basically identical results, despite the well-known fact that the whole algae are not digestible due to the very hard outer shell. A rat study also using the whole algae found a decrease of some tumor cell markers in hepatocellular carcinoma model, but the daily dose was around 20–30 g for a normal size human (Arifin et al., 2017). Another older study showed increased antitumor immunity after supplementation with a *Chlorella* diet reaching 10%. Detailed investigation revealed that these effects were mediated via increased T lymphocyte action (Tanaka et al., 1990).

An interesting study found that oral supplementation with heavy doses increased aerobic endurance capacity in young individuals. Due to the low number of participants and heterogeneous training history among participants, this study needs to be repeated before any meaningful conclusion can be made.

Another species, *Chlorella pyrenoidosa*, was used for evaluation of the effects in people suffering from fibromyalgia, hypertension, and ulcerative colitis. The results showed slight improvements in all aspects. There are, however, problems associated with this study. First, the participants had to take two different *Chlorella* supplements, so we do not know which one was the active material. And, second, it was necessary to take an extremely high daily dose of 10 g (i.e., 50 tablets) plus 100 mL of extract (Merchant and Andre, 2001). The same group later continued with somehow lower doses, but the results evaluating the effects of 2-month supplementation on blood pressure showed only minimal effects.

There is an increasing concern regarding the use of *Chlorella* in humans, and its various molecules with antigenic features, which are also seen in infectious microorganisms. Some studies found lipopolysaccharide-like molecules (Armstrong et al., 2002), which are likely to provoke inflammation; others found phosphoglycans resembling the virulence factors of *Leishmania* (Suarez et al., 2010).

Chlorella can contain substantial levels of iodine, and people with iodine sensitive thyroid conditions or iodine allergies should avoid using it. Some people can have direct allergy to *Chlorella*, manifesting in rashes or itching. The high content of vitamin K could interfere with blood clotting abilities. Another study showed that nausea, abdominal pain, and skin rash were among the most often reported adverse reactions. In addition, preexisting medical conditions, namely renal failure and hypothyroidism, were associated with increased occurrence of side effects (Rzymski and Jaskiewicz, 2017).

A rather negative study regarding the use of *Chlorella* in mice with mammary tumors clearly demonstrated that supplementation with 200 mg/kg promoted the growth of tumors, probably by creating a protumor microenvironment (Khalilnezhad et al., 2018).

As some studies reported interesting effects of *Chlorella* supplementation, it is important to remember that, in all cases, very high doses were necessary, often making its use under normal conditions rather impractical and difficult. The rather high amount of potentially dangerous side effects clearly shows that we need to be really careful before any decision about using *Chlorella* as a supplement is made.

References

An, H.J., Rim, H.K., Jeong, H.J., Hong, S.H., Um, J.Y., Kim, H.M.: Hot water extracts of *Chlorella vulgaris* improve immune function in protein-deficient weanling mice and immune cells. Immunopharmacol. Immunotoxicol., 32: 585-592, 2010.

Arifin, K.T., Sulaiman, S., Saad, S.M., Damanhuri, H.A., Ngah, W.Z.W., Yusof, Y.A.M.: Evaluation of tumour markers TGF-b, M_2-PK, OV-6 and AFP in hepatocellular carcinoma (HCC)-induced rats and their suppression by microalgae *Chlorella vulgaris*. BMC Cancer, 17, 2017, doi:10.1186/s12885-017-3883-3.

Armstrong, P.B., Armstrong, M.T., Pardy, R.I., Child, A., Wainwright, N.: Immunohistochemical demonstration of a lipopolysaccharide in the cell wall of a eukaryote, the green algae, *Chlorella*. Biol. Bull., 203: 203-204, 2002.

Bae, M.J., Shin, H.S., Chai, O.H., Han, J.G., Shon, D.H.: Inhibitory effect of unicellular green algae (*Chlorella vulgaris*) water extract on allergic immune response. J. Sci. Food. Agric., 93: 3133-3136, 2013.

de Souza Queiroz, J., Barbosa, C.M.V., da Rocha, M.C., Bincoletto, C., Paredes-Gamero, E.J., de Souza Queiroz, M.L., Neto, J.P.: *Chlorella vulgaris* treatment ameliorates the suppressive effects of single and repeated stressors on hematopoieses. Brain, Behavior, Immun., 20: 39-50, 2016.

Justo, G.Z., Silva, M.R., Queiroz, M.L.: Effects of the green algae *Chlorella vulgaris* on the response of the host hematopoietic system to intraperitoneal Ehrlich ascites tumor transplantation in mice. Immunopharmacol. Immunotoxicol., 23: 119-132, 2001.

Kang, H., Lee, C.H., Kim, J.R., Kwon, J.Y., Seo, S.G., Han, J.G., Kim, B.G., Kim, J.E., Lee, K.W.: *Chlorella vulgaris* attenuates *Dermatophagoides farinae*-induced atopic dermatitis-like syndromes in NC/Nga mice. Int. J. Mol. Sci., 16: 21021-21034, 2015.

Kay, R.A.: Microalgae as food and supplement. Crit. Rev. Food Sci. Nutrit., 30: 555-573, 1991.

Khalilnezhad, A., Mahmoudian, E., Mosaffa, N., Anissian, A.: Effects of *Chlorella vulgaris* on tumor gworth in mammary tumor-bearing Balb/c mice: discussing association of an immune-suppressed protumor microenvironment with serum IFNγ and IgG decrease and spleen IgG potentiation. Eur. J. Nutr., 57: 1025-1044, 2018.

Kwak, J.H., Baek, S.H., Woo, Y., Han, J.K., Kim, B.G., Kim, O.Y., Lee, J.H.: Beneficial immunostimulatory effect of short-term *Chlorella* supplementation: enhancement of natural killer cell activity and early inflammatory response (randomized, double-blinded, placebo-controlled trial). Nutr. J., 11, 2012, doi:10.1186/1475-2891-11-53.

Lin, P.Y., Tsai, C.AT., Chuang, L.W., Chao, Y.H., Pan, I.H., Chen, Y.K., Lin, C.C., Wang, B.Y. *Chlorella sorokiniana* induces mitochondrial-mediated apoptosis in human non-small cell lung cancer cells and inhibits xenograft tumor growth in vivo. BMC Complement. Alt. Med., 17, 2017, doi:10.1186/s12906-017-0611-9.

Merchant, R.E., Andre, C.A.: A review of recent clinical trials of the nutritional supplement *Chlorella pyrenoidosa* in the treatment of fibromyalgia, hypertension, and ulcerative colitis. Alt. Therap., 7: 79-90, 2001.

Muyazawa, Y., Murayama, T., Goya, N., Wang, L.F., Tung, Y.C., Yamagucho, N.: Immunomodulation by a unicellular green algae (*Chlorella pyrenoidosa*) in tumor bearing mice. J. Ethnopharmacol., 24: 135-146, 1988.

Otsuki, T., Shimizu, K., Lemitsu, M., Kono, I.L.: Salivary secretory immunoglobulin a secretion increases after 4-weeks ingestion of chlorella-derived multicomponent supplement in humans: a randomized cross over study. Nutr. J., 10, 2011, doi:10.1186/1475-2891-10-91.

Panahi, Y., Darvishi, B., Jowzi, N., Beiraghdar, F., Sahebkar, A.: *Chlorella vulgaris* - a multifunctional dietary supplement with diverse medicinal properties. Curr. Pharmacol. Design, 22: 164-173, 2016.

Rzynski, P., Jaskiewicz, M.: Microalgal food supplements from the perspective of Polish consumers: patterns of use, adverse events, and beneficial effects. J. Appl. Phycol., 29:1841-1850, 2017, doi:10.1007/s10811-017-1079-5.

Suarez, E.R., Kralovec, J.A., Grindley T.B.: Isolation of phosphorylated polysaccharides from algae: the immunostimulatory principle of *Chlorella pyrenoidosa*. Carbohydr. Res., 345: 1190-1204, 2010.

Tanaka, K., Tomita, Y., Tauruta, M., Konishi, F., Himeno, F., Nomoto, K.: Oral administration of *Chlorella vulgaris* augments concomitant antitumor immunity. Immunopharmacol., 12: 277-291, 1990.

6

ELDERBERRY

Black elderberry (*Sambucus nigra*) is one of the oldest medicinal plants noted for its cardiovascular, anti-inflammatory, and immune-stimulatory properties. Extracts of the elderberry have been used by Native Americans as a natural remedy against fever and rheumatism. In Europe, it is often called a "natural antibiotic," as it contains high levels of three bioflavonoids: kaempferol, quercetin, and anthocyanin. Several versions of elderflower drink recipes can be traced back to the Roman period. Ancient Egyptians used it to improve their complexions and heal burns. In the United States, the plant has been called "the medicine chest of country people." In many European regions, elderberry syrup is prepared at home and consumed daily. Besides flowers, other parts of the bush are commonly used including berries (Figure 5) and bark. In folk medicine, juice or even dried berries are used to treat influenza, various infections, sciatica, toothache, and headaches as well as used as a laxative and diuretic. In addition, berries are a low-calorie food full of vitamins and dietary fiber. The major health benefits are, however, ascribed to the fact they are packed with antioxidants.

Out of many *Sambucus* species, *S. nigra* is mostly used. American elderberry (*S. canadensis*) is much less studied. A comparative study found more anthocyanins in the American elderberry and some bioactivity relevant to inhibition of both the initiation and promotion stages of carcinogenesis

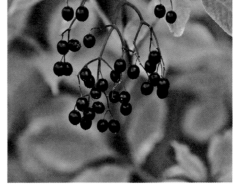

Figure 5 Berries of elderberry

(Thole et al., 2006). This study, however, used mouse epidermal cell line instead of the usual panel of cancer cell lines. It measured reduction in some enzymes instead of direct effects on cancer *in vivo*, making the claims rather unclear.

The problem with elderberry extract is similar to problems of other plant-derived immunomodulators: several different species of *Sambucus* are used for preparation of supplement, without considering that their anthocyanin and phenolic profiles are substantially different. A study comparing biological effects of elderberry juices (obtained from eight different genotypes) found that only one juice had anti-oxidant properties (Jiang et al., 2015). To further complicate the situation, both ethanol, acetone, and water extractions are used. Whereas chromatographic patterns are similar, levels of individual compounds differ between the extractions. The anti-oxidant activity fully correlated with total phenolic content. Readers seeking more details on individual compositions should see a comparative study of Mikulic-Petkovsek et al. (2015). The exact nutritional composition of elderberries depends on variety, ripeness and climatic and environmental conditions. A detailed study comparing different types of extraction found significant differences in content of phenolic constituents. A detailed study measured the content of polyphenols, organic acids, and sugars among diverse elderberry genotypes grown in three Missouri locations. The results showed significant differences in all tested parameters among sites, genotypes, and years (Thomas et al., 2015).

Anthocyanins are a major group of naturally occurring substances belonging to the flavonoid family particularly anthocyanins, flavonoids, and other polyphenols. Besides being responsible for the attractive colors, anthocyanins are potent antioxidants. It is important to note that besides bioactive compounds in food, bioavailability including metabolism and excretion is critical, too. Recent studies showed that bioavailability of anthocyanin metabolites is 42-fold higher than parent anthocyanin. In addition, encapsulation of anthocyanins in liposomes or microparticles further increased availability.

Several clinical trials showed some symptoms of the influenza infection, such as sneezing and fever, rapidly recovered after treatment with elderberry juice (Zakay-Rones et al., 2004). A detailed study evaluated anti-influenza virus effects of elderberry juice and its fraction. It found strong *in vivo* effects of the juice and its fractions. From these results, we can conclude that despite strong differences in levels of anthocyanins and polyphenols, the antiviral action was similar to the full juice (Kinoshita et al., 2012). A recent detailed review of the antiviral properties of elderberry products found that the lack of real studies comparing these products with standard anti-viral medications makes informed and detailed recommendations of elderberry extract use in medical application impractical (Porter and Bode, 2017). A double-blind placebo-controlled clinical trial showed that elderberry supplementation reduced cold duration and symptoms in air-travelers (Tiralongo et al., 2016). Besides the effect on colds and influenza, elderberry extracts were reported to be effective in stimulating immune responses by enhancing production and secretion of cytokines by monocytes.

Studies of the possible effects on the heart are contradictory. Some studies suggested possible reduction of fat in blood and a decrease of cholesterol levels, but other studies found no effects at all. Elderberry fruit fractions have anti-inflammatory activity. An animal study showed that the addition of elderberry extract attenuated fish oil–induced hyperlipidemia and oxidative stress (Dubey et al., 2012). Not only did this study confirm antioxidant effects, but suggested fish oil is co-supplemented with anthocyanin-rich elderberry extract. This might allow for the positive effects of fish oil supplementation without the negative effects. Anti-oxidants disarm free radicals; therefore, decreasing tissue and cardiovascular damage. In this regard, the anti-oxidant capacity for elderberry is among the highest measured in fruits and berries. It is important to remember, however, that despite laboratory proof of strong anti-oxidant capacities, the direct proof that dietary anti-oxidant phytochemicals can reduce human disease by inhibiting *in vivo* oxidative processes has been elusive. This is mostly because the amount of bioavailable anti-oxidant is low and not delivered at the place of harmful oxidative processes.

Like with all natural plant-derived material, there is no standardized method for measuring the number of bioactive components, like anthocyanins, in commercial products. The levels mentioned on the label will depend on the method used for measurements. It is important to note that bark, unripe berries, and seeds contain small amounts of cyanogenic glycosides, but potential health hazards will disappear after cooking. However, raw berries also contain low levels of lectin, which can enter the circulation after oral uptake and can play a role in inducing the so-called early IL-4 formation involved in stimulation of allergic reactions (Haas et al. 1999).

To conclude, it is clear that the use of elderberry, particularly in juice form, has reported some benefits such as reduction of cholesterol levels, improvements after infections and as oxidants. While the results are interesting, further research is needed not only to confirm these possibilities in better controlled experiments, but also to elucidate the possible mechanisms of such effects. So far, there is only limited evidence for any health claims. Besides reduction of length and severity of flu symptoms, elderberry cannot be recommended for any particular health benefit and might better serve as a healthy and colorful component of our diet.

References

Dubey, P., Jayasooriya, A.P., Cheema, S.K.: Fish oil induced hyperlipidemia and oxidative stress in BioF1B hamsters is attenuated by elderberry extract. Appl. Physiol. Nutr. Metab., 37: 472-479, 2012.

Haas, H., Falcone, F.H., Schramm, G., Halsch, K., Gibbs, B.F., Klaucke, J., Poppelmann, M., Becker, W.M., Gabius, H.J., Schlaak, M.: Dietary lectins can induce *in vitro* release of IL-4 and IL-13 from human basophils. Eur. J. Immunol., 29: 918-827, 1999.

Jiang, J.M., Zong, Y., Chuang, D.Y., Lei, W., Lu, C.H., Gu, Z., Fritche, K.L., Thomas, A.L., Lubahn, D.B., Simonyi, A., Sun, G.Y.: Effects of elderberry juice from different genotypes on oxidative and inflammatory responses in microglial cells. Acta Hortic., 1061: 281-288, 2015.

Kinoshita, E., Hayashi, K., Katayama, H., Hausahi, T., Obata, A.: Anti-influenza virus effects of elderberry juice and its fraction. Biosci. Biotechnol. Biochem., 76: 1633-1638, 2012.

Mikulic-Petkovsek, M., Samoticha, J., Eler, K., Stampar, F., Verebic, R.: Traditional elderflower beverages: A rich source of phenolic compounds with high antioxidant activity. J. Agricult. Food Chem., 63: 1477-1487, 2015.

Porter, R.S., Bode, R.F.: A review of the antiviral properties of black elder (*Sambucus nigra* L.) products. Phytother. Res., 31: 533-554, 2017.

Thole, J.M., Burns Kraft, T.F., Sueiro, L.A., Kang, Y.H., Gills, J.J., Cuendet, M., Pezzuto, J.M., Seigler, D.S., Lila, M.A.: A comparative evaluation of the anticancer properties of European and American elderberry fruits. J. Med. Food, 9: 498-504, 2006.

Thomas, A.I., Byers, P.L., Gu, S., Avery, J.D., Datta, A.,Fernando, L., Grossi, P., Rottinghaus, G.E.: Occurrence of polyphenols, organic acids and sugars among diverse elderberry genotypes grown in three Missouri (USA) locations. Acta Hortic., 1061: 147-154, 2015.

Tiralongo, E., Wee, S.S., Lea, R.A.: Elderberry supplementation reduces cold duration and symptoms in air travelers: A randomized, double-blind placebo-controlled clinical trials. Nutrients, 8, 2016, doi:10.3390/nu8040182.

Zakay-Rones, Z., Thom, E., Wollan, AT., Wadstein, J.: Randomized study of the efficacy and safety of oral elderberry extract in the treatment of influenza A and B virus infections. J. Int. Med. Res., 32: 132-140, 2004.

7

ELLAGIC ACID

Ellagic acid is a polyphenol found in a wide variety of vegetables and fruits (i.e., cranberries, pomegranates, raspberries, strawberries, and peaches). Some studies estimate that in fruits like strawberries, ellagic acid comprises up to 51% of the phenolic compounds. Walnuts represent another source, as their main polyphenol is pedunculagin, an ellagitannin, which after consumption is hydrolyzed to release ellagic acid. Ellagic acid is a dimeric derivative of gallic acid and rarely occurs free in diet crops, but is usually conjugated with glycosides or forms part of ellagitannins. Readers seeking detailed information on the chemical structure (Figure 6) and metabolism of ellagitannins should read the excellent review by Lipinska et al. (2014). The bioavailability of ellagitannins and free ellagic acid depends on the part of gastrointestinal tract in which these compounds are absorbed, as they are stable under the acidic gastric environment.

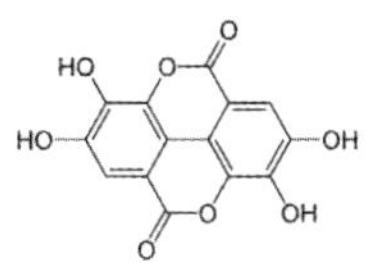

Figure 6   Chemical structure of ellagic acid

Some studies have reported anti-oxidant, anti-diabetic, anti-proliferative, and anti-carcinogenic properties. Antimicrobial and immunomodulating effects showed increased levels of specific antibodies in an *Aeromonas* infection model (Abuelsaad et al., 2013), suggesting a possible role in inhibition, or at least reduction, of infections. The authors concluded that ellagic acid worked as a strong adjuvant. Walnut polyphenols were shown to have some biological activities, but mostly *in vitro*, which is still a far cry from their use as supplement. For example, the finding that adding ellagic acid increases *in vitro* anti-bacterial effects of antibiotics is more or less scientific exercise, because, for any practical use, you need to use oral supplementation *in vivo*.

One of the few studies evaluating the effects of long-term supplementation with doses from 0.5 - 2 mg/kg/day revealed that this sub chronic exposure significantly suppressed specific antibody formation and cytotoxic function of T lymphocytes. All other immunological parameters remained unchanged (Allen et al., 2003). These data raised an important question about the possible side effects in using ellagic acid not only in immunocompromised patients, but also in healthy people.

A unique study found *in vitro* inhibition of HIV-1 infection without any cytotoxicity (Promsong et al., 2018), which, if confirmed, might lead to the development of a novel microbicide against HIV-1 infection. It is important to note, however, that the authors used 95% pure chemical ellagic acid, and not any of the commercial extracts.

Oral administration of purified ellagic acid alleviated radiation-induced and aluminium chloride–induced liver damage (Salem et al., 2016). Some studies suggested inhibition of alcohol-induced liver damage via an increase of anti-oxidant levels. The amount of pure ellagic acid is, however, rather high and represents at least 5 g/day (Devipriya et al., 2007). A study on fish found improved hematological, immunological, and anti-oxidant parameters, but again, the necessary dose was rather high. Similarly, hydrolysable tannins are phenolic phytochemicals with high anti-oxidant and free radical scavenging activities. As with most anti-oxidants, they are highly active *in vitro*, but almost worthless *in vivo* (Larrosa et al., 2010).

Another study evaluated the effects of oral supplementation with ellagic acid on experimentally-induced hepatitis. The results showed significant improvements and the mechanisms of action probably involve Toll-like receptors and protein-kinase/nuclear factor kB signaling pathway (Lee et al., 2014).

Other reports showed that administration of ellagic acid reduced the level of lipids in circulation and lowered the elevation of plasma cholesterol. A study testing the effects of ellagic acid in arsenic-trioxide–induced cardiotoxicity found rather interesting results, as it showed that ellagic acid pretreatment significantly ameliorated cardiotoxicity, most probably via its anti-oxidant properties.

Dietary phenols in general have received attention for their ability to modulate lipid and glucose metabolism. In addition to the health benefits from flavonoids, it is also notable that several nonflavonoid polyphenolic compounds are considered to be important for metabolic health. Ellagic acid seems to have an antidiabetic activity through the action on b-cells of pancreas, stimulating insulin secretion and decreasing glucose intolerance. Treatment with an extract rich in ellagic acid has been reported to significantly decrease fasting glucose levels in diabetic animals and increased serum insulin levels.

A detailed review of the effects of ellagic acid in metabolic health is given by Kang et al. (2016). The authors summarize how intake of ellagic acid regulates lipid metabolism, and delineate the potential mechanisms of action on obesity-mediated metabolic complications. The results suggest that ellagic acid is a modulator of the gut microbiome and serves as an epigenetic effector. A detailed study found that food supplementation significantly improved metabolic syndrome caused by a high-carbohydrate, high-fat diet (Panchal et al., 2012). The problem, however, is that to see these results, the animals had to consume extreme doses of ellagic acid, equivalent to 56 g/day for a normal adult person. Recommending the inclusion of ellagic acid–containing fruits and nuts in the diet may be a promising strategy to lessen adiposity and to improve obesity-related metabolic complication.

Various experimental models of ulcerative colitis showed that supplementation with ellagic acid ameliorated disease severity of acute model and inhibited the disease progression in chronic model. The data suggested that these effects manifested via the anti-inflammatory effects of ellagic acid. Similar data were later found in Crohn disease. Using an unrelated model, anti-inflammatory activity was found in rats.

Using pomegranate extracts rich in ellagic acid, scientist found reduction of oxidative stress and platelet aggregation, inhibition of lipid uptake by macrophages, reduction of blood glucose levels, and regulation of blood pressure. Clinical studies demonstrated suppression of hypertension and attenuation of atherosclerosis; for review, see Wang et al. (2018). A rat study of the anti-oxidant effects against skeletal muscle ischemia injury revealed some improvements after oral administration of ellagic acid (Akdemir et al., 2016). It is important to note that this study used a purified ellagic acid and not a commercial extract.

Most studies do not use an isolated component, but instead use an extract rich in various phenols including ellagic acid. Despite the fact that the results are often interesting, they do not allow any conclusion about which molecule is responsible. That alone represents a significant problem, because biological extracts notoriously differ from one batch to another. A study reporting the immunosuppressive effects of extracts of *Phyllanthus amarus* (Ilangkovan et al., 2015) is particularly interesting and allows us to reach several conclusions. On one hand, it offers the possibility of using the extract for patients needing to suppress their immune reactions (such as after transplantation or with serious autoimmune disease); on the other hand, it suggests potential problems due to unwanted suppression of defense reactions. This leaves us wondering which of the many bioactive substances present in the mixture is really responsible for the effects. This is an extremely important point––individual fruits, pomegranate in particular, often provide various and important health benefits. Recent observations suggested that the molecules responsible for the nutritional and health benefits of pomegranate might not be ellagic acid but urolithins. However, our current knowledge does not allow us to contribute these benefits to any particular component of the fruits.

A human study found that pomegranate ellagotannins have positive effects on growth of *Lacrobacillus* and *Bifidobacterium* in gut, suggesting the potential role as prebiotics. Using experimentally-induced model of gastric ulceration, oral administration of ellagic acid showed gastroprotective and ulcer-healing properties, probably via increase in the nitric oxide production (Beserra et al., 2011). The most interesting conclusion of this study was the fact that when the authors tested three different inductions of ulceration, the effects of supplementation were similar, but the mechanisms were different in each model. In general, the effects were mediated by strengthening the defensive factors and attenuating the offensive factors. The anti-ulcer activity and possible healing mechanisms were even higher when ellagic acid was used together with gallic acid.

Another potentially important bioactive metabolite is isourolithin A, which can be produced from ellagic acid by the action of intestinal bacteria. This ability, however, differs considerably among individuals depending on their gut microbiota composition (Selma et al., 2017). Isolation and characterization of the specific bacteria may be useful in preparation of new probiotics.

An interesting study demonstrated that the combination of

ellagic acid and curcumin had solid anti-cancer properties against cervical carcinoma (Kumar et al., 2016). This study, however, suffers from two major problems: first, it uses only cervical cancer cell line, HeLa, and no other control (cancerous or negative) cell line, so we do not know if these results are unique for cervical cancer or for any cancer (not to mention for any cell in culture). And second, the testing is done *in vitro*, which might and might not be relevant to the situation *in vivo*. The problems with using cell lines was further underlined in a study showing that ellagic acid induced concentration-dependent Ca^{2+} rise in HepG2 human hepatoma cells, but not in the additional three hepatoma cell lines tested. In addition, ellagic acid caused death of all human hepatoma cell lines, but not mouse hepatocytes (Liang et al., 2016). The authors of the study did not explain the possible reasons for this discrepancy, making some of the *in vitro* studies of the natural bioactive molecules questionable.

Anti-tumor activity was, similar to most natural immunomodulators, established mostly on cell lines. The best results were found when ellagic acid was not used in extract form, but was directly synthesized. The rare *in vivo* experiments showed anti-cancer properties against esophageal cancer, probably via inhibition of some carcinogenic substances and/or by limiting the mutagenic properties of some chemical compounds (Lipinska et al., 2014). Another study demonstrated using a *Sanguisorba officinalis* extract rich in ellagic acid could arrest cell cycle and induce mitochondrial pathway apoptosis in cancer cells *in vitro*. Oral uptake of the same extract resulted in significant reduction of breast cancer growth (Wang et al., 2012). Rather controversial results were obtained in a study using newborn mice pretreated with ellagic acid before receiving an injection of the carcinogen. Depending on the chemical, the data showed either significant reduction of lung tumors or no effects at all. Similar experiments found 25–50% inhibition of the development of chemically-induced esophageal cancer, but only when the ellagic acid was used continuously before, during, and after the chemical treatment. If used as a treatment, ellagic acid showed no effects (Mandal and Stoner, 1990). The possible mechanisms by which ellagic acid may inhibit cancer development are given in a comprehensive review by Hannum (2004).

An interesting study examined effects of ellagic acid on cognitive impairments, particularly long-term potentiation deficits and brain inflammation in animals with traumatic brain injury. The data revealed significant effects of oral administration in preventing brain inflammation and cognitive deficits (Farbood et al., 2015).

A comparative study of phytochemical composition of numerous commercial pomegranate-based products produced in 11 countries showed that the ranges of punicalagin and ellagic acid contents were 0.96 to 308 mg/g and 0.09 to 13.1 mg/g, respectively, showing the differences between the labeling and reality (Cano-Lamadrid et al., 2017).

In summary, ellagic acid seems to have some interesting biological properties, but better characterized extracts are needed.

References

Abuelsaad, A.S.A., Mohamed, I., Allam, G., Al-Solumani, A.A.: Antimicrobial and immunomodulating activities of hesperidin and ellagic acid against diarrheic *Aeromonas hydrophila* in a murine model. Life Sci., 93: 714-722, 2013.

Akdemir, F.N.E., Gulcin, I., Karagox, B., Soslu, R., Alwasel, S.H.: A comparative study on the antioxidant effects of hesperidin and ellagic acid against skeletal muscle ischemia/reperfusion injury. J. Enzyme Inhib. Med. Chem., 31: 114-118, 2016.

Allen, C.T., Peden-Adams, M.M., EuDaly, J., Kell, D.E.: Subchronic exposure to ellagic acid impairs cytotoxic T-cell function and suppresses humoral immunity in mice. Immunopharmacol. Immunotoxicol., 25: 409-423, 2003.

Bessera, A.M.S.S., Calegari, P.I., Souza, M.C., dos Santos, R.A.N., da Silva Lima, J.C., Silva, R.M., Balogun, S.O., de Oliveira Martins, D.T.: Gastroprotective and ulcer-healing mechanisms of ellagic acid in experimental rats. J. Agric. Food. Chem., 59: 6957-6965, 2011.

Cano-Lamadrid, M., Lipan, L., Calin-Sanchez, A., Hernandez, F., Carbonell-Barrachina, A.A.: A comparative study between labeling and reality: The case of phytochemical composition of commercial pmegranate-based products. J. Food Sci., 82: 1820-1826, 2017.

Devipriya, N., Srinivasan, M., Sudheer, A.A.R., Menon, V.P.: Effect of ellagic acid, a natural polyphenol, on alcohol-induced prooxidant and antioxidant imbalance: a drug dose dependent study. Singapore Med., 48: 311-318, 2007.

Farbood, Y., Sarkaki, A., Dianat, M., Khodadadi, A., Haddad, M.K., Mashadizadeh, S.: Ellagic acid prevents cognitive and hippocampal long-term potentiation deficits and brain inflammation in rat with traumatic brain injury. Life Sci., 124: 120-127, 2015.

Hannum, S.M.: Potential impact of strawberries on human health: A review of the science. Crit. Rev. Food Sci. Nutr., 44: 1-17, 2004.

Ilangkovan, M., Jantan, I., Mesail, M.A., Bukhari, S.N.A.: Immunosuppressive effects of the standardized extract of *Phyllanthus amarus* on cellular immune responses in Wistar-Kyoto rats. Drug Design Dev. Therap., 9: 4917-4930, 2015.

Kang, I., Bruckner, T., Shay, N.F., Chung, S.: Improvements in metabolic health with consumption of ellagic acid and subsequent conversion into urolithins: Evidence and mechanisms. Adv. Nutr., 7: 961-967, 2016.

Kumar, D., Basu, S., Parija, L., Rout, D., Manna, S., Dandapat, J., Debata, P.R.: Curcumin and ellagic acid synergistically induce ROS generation, DNA damage, p53 accumulation and apoptosis in HeLa cervical carcinoma cells. Biomed. Pharmacotherap., 81: 31-37, 2016.

Larrosa, M., Garcia-Conesa, M.T., Espin, J.C., Tomas-Barbelan, F.A.: Ellagitannins, ellegic acid and vascular health. Mol. Asp. Med., 31: 513-530, 2010.

Lee, J.H., Won, J.H., Choi, J.M., Cha, H., Jang, Y.J., Park, S., Kim, H.G., Kim, H.C., Kim, D.K.: Protective effect of ellagic acid on Concanavalin A-induced hepatitis via Toll-like receptor and mitogen-activated protein kinase/nuclear kB signaling pathways. J. Agric. Food Chem., 62: 10110-10117, 2014.

Liang, W.Z., Chou, C.T., Cheng, J.S., Wang, J.L., Chang, H.T., Chen, I.S., Lu, T., Yeh, J.H., Kuo, D.H., Shieh, P., Chen, F.A., Kuo, C.C., Jan, C.R.: The effect of the phenol compound ellagic acid on Ca^{2+} homeostasis and cytotoxicity in liver cells. Eur. J. Pharmacol., 780: 243-251, 2016.

Lipinska, L., Klewicka, E., Sojka, M.: Structure, occurrence and biological activity of ellagitannins: A general review. Acta Sci. Pol. Technol. Aliment., 13: 289-299, 2014.

Mandal, S., Stoner, G.D.: Inhibition of N-nitrosobenzyl-methylamine-induced esophageal tumorigenesis in rats by ellagic acid. Carcinogenesis, 11: 55-61, 1990.

Panchal, S.K., Ward, L., Brown, L.: Ellagic acid attenuates high-carbohydrate, high-fat diet-induced metabolic syndrome in rats. Eur. J. Nutr., 52: 559-568, 2012.

Promsong, A., Chuenchitra, T., Saipin, K., Tewtrakul, S., Panichayupakaranant, P., Satthakarn, S., Nittayananta, W.: Ellagic acid inhibits HIV-1 infection *in vitro:* Potential role as a novel microbicide. Oral Dis., 24: 249-252, 2018.

Salem, A.M., Mohammaden, T.F., Ali, M.A.M., Mohamed, E.A., Hasan, H.F.: Ellagic and ferulic acids alleviate radiation and aluminium chloride-induced oxidative damage. Life Sci., 160: 2-11, 2016.

Selma, M.V., Beltran, D., Luna, M.C., Romo-Vaquero, M., Garcia-Villalba, R., Mira, A., Espin, J.C., Tomas-Barberan, F.A.T.: Isolation of human intestinal bacterial capable of producing bioactive metabolite isourolithin A from ellagic acid. Frontiers Microbiol., 2017, doi:10/3389/fmicb.2017.01521.

Wang, D., Ozen, C., Abu-Reidah, I.M., Chigurupati, S., Patra, J.K., Horbanczuk, J.O., Jozwik, A., Tzvetkov, N.T., Uhrin, P., Atanasov, A.G.: Vacruloprotective effects of pomegranate (*Punica granatum* L.). Frontiers Pharmacol., 2018, doi:10.3398/fpahr.2018.00544.

Wang, Z.Y., Loo, W.T.Y., Wang, N., Chow, L.W.C., Wang, D., Han, F., Zheng, X., Chen, J.P.: Effect of *Sanguisorba officinalis* L. on breast cancer growth and angiogenesis. Exp. Opin. Therapeut. Targets, 16: S79-S89, 2012.

8

ESSENTIAL OILS

Essential oils are volatile liquid substances extracted from aromatic plant material by steam distillation or mechanical expression. These oils are traditionally used in perfumery, cosmetics, and food. Oils produced with the aid of chemical solvents are not considered true essential oils.

Essential oils are often used in aromatherapy, usually for the improvement of physical, emotional, and spiritual well-being. The typical form of usage is inhalation and topical treatment. In some cases, however, these oils are ingested. The results of aromatherapy are theorized to result from binding of released chemical components present in essential oil to receptors in the olfactory bulb; thus, subsequently impacting the limbic system. Topical application is supposed to have antibacterial, anti-inflammatory, and analgesic effects.

Plant essential oils are reservoirs of bioactive molecules. They are complex mixtures of volatile and lipophilic organic substances synthesized as secondary metabolites. These oils are isolated mainly by distillation and pressing. They consist of dozens and sometimes even hundreds of individual components, which include monoterpenes, esters, alcohols, ketones, phenols, and aldehydes. A single study on one essential oil found 74 potentially bioactive molecules in significant quantities and another 34 compounds in trace amounts. Most are volatile and responsible for the characteristic odor.

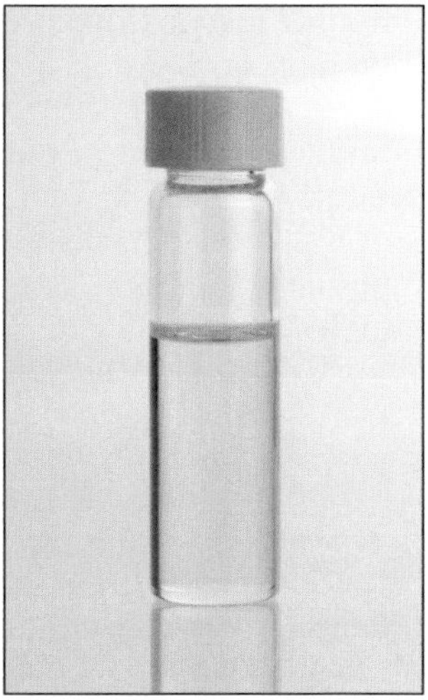

Figure 7 Essential oil

Another study found a total of 85 components; 70 components in oils from normal roots and 65 components in oils from hairy roots of the same plant.

Antioxidant food supplements may be used to help our body reduce oxidative damage caused by free radicals produced both in normal and pathological cell metabolism. Oxidative enzymes, such as superoxide dismutase, usually protect our organisms, but when the process of antioxidant protection becomes unbalanced, problems with physiological functions might result in various diseases and accelerated aging. Therefore, a significant push to study potentially naturally-occurring anti-oxidants has been made in recent years. A comparative evaluation of the anti-oxidant properties of 248 essential oils revealed that only 7% had high oxidative activity, which was connected to the presence of oxygenated monoterpenoids and monoterpene phenols (Saleh et al., 2010). Some of these effects might be due to the inhibition of neutrophil responses.

A mouse study evaluated the effects of essential oils on experimentally-induced acute airway inflammation and found significant improvements via inhibition of IL-13 production and Th immune responses.

Linalool (coriander essential oil) has some anti-tumorigenic potential via modulation of oxidative stress. A comparative study showed that clove essential oil enhanced delayed-type hypersensitivity response and restored chemotherapy-damaged cellular and humoral immune responses. Other essential oils recovered only humoral immunity or had no activity at all. Cinnamon essential oil had some anti-inflammatory activity. Clove essential oil and extracts showed immunomodulatory and anti-inflammatory action on cytokine production by macrophages. Marigold oil has anti-oxidative and anti-inflammatory effects; whereas, parsley essential oil suppressed immune response. A comparative study testing 15 different essential oils found significant inhibition of phagocytosis, suggesting a suppression of at least natural immunity (Perez-Roses et al., 2015).

Possible effects of inhibiting cancer growth are summarized in a recent review by Blowman et al. (2018). Most studies evaluated only *in vitro* effects on various cancer cells, ranging from breast to prostate cancer. Each of the studies used either essential oil derived from different species, used different cancer cell line, or found a different mechanism of action. Oils from roots of *Leonurus sibiricus* had anti-bacterial, anti-inflammatory, anti-oxidant and anti-cancer properties.

The study was done *in vitro* only and the effects were observed in high doses only (Sitarek et al., 2017). Some of the oils were found to have direct toxic effects on cancer cells, but most of their biological activities were manifested via positive effects on the immune system. It is likely that the activity of the main components of essential oils was modulated by other minor molecules. In this case, it might be better to use whole essential oils rather than its isolated components.

In some reports, essential oils had little or even no effects (Villarini et al., 2014). For a recent review of anti-cancer activity of essential oils, see Bhalla et al. (2013). Although many studies reported possible mechanisms of action for essential oil compounds, no consensus has been reached (Andrade et al., 2018). The use of highly purified oils (i.e., ~98%) showed much better immunostimulating effects (Farhath et al., 2013). Some reports stated the responsible molecule is carvacrol, which was found to have anticancer properties in various preclinical models of carcinoma, acting on pro-apoptotic processes. Clearly, more studies are necessary in order to apply them safely and appropriately; so far no clinical trials on carvacrol exist.

Another possible application are infections. Whereas direct anti-bacterial effects or decreases in infection severity are limited, some essential oils seem to have synergetic effects when used simultaneously with antibiotics. Even as these reports suggest only moderate synergism, with constantly increasing threat of antibody resistance, this possibility clearly needs more studies to evaluate possible mechanisms of action; for review, see Tangeveld et al. (2014). Significant attention has been focused on use of essential oils as potential anti-microbials to treat skin diseases. At least 90 essential oils have been identified that can be recommended for dermatological use. However, these oils are rarely used directly, as direct use onto the skin can cause irritation (Harding, 2002). Therefore, essential oils are blended with carrier oils, which might be partly responsible for the biological effects. Recent comprehensive reviews of commercial essential oils in dermatology found some effects but the combination, dosing, and possible resistance are still unknown (Orchard and van Vuuren, 2017). Oregano oil was found to have bactericidal properties against various multidrug-resistant clinical isolates both *in vivo* and *in vitro*, without having any irritating effects (Lu et al., 2018). Carvacrol, a phenolic monoterpenoid found in numerous essential oils, might be the molecule responsible for significant anti-microbial activity; for review, see Sharifi-Rad et al. (2017).

In our own research, we focused on the biological effects of thymus (thyme) essential oils. We compared seven different thymus-derived essential oils. First, we focused on their chemical composition, followed by testing their effects on phagocytosis, cytokine production, chemotaxis, edema inhibition, and liver protection. We found limited biological activities among tested oils, with no correlation between composition and biological effects. Similarly, no oils were effective on every reaction. Based on our data, the biological use of these essential oils is questionable (Vetvicka and Vetvickova, 2016). In conclusion, the present study found that essential oils isolated from thyme have some biological activities on chemotaxis, IL-1b and IL-6 production, and on reduction of experimentally-induced liver damage. These oils had no effects on cell proliferation or phagocytosis. At the same time, none of these oils showed superior effects. Compared to another popular natural immunomodulator, b-glucan, these biological effects were very limited (Vetvicka and Vetvickova, 2010). Similar results reached a comparative study of nine commercial essential oils (Al-Tamini et al., 2016).

Individual essential oils differ in suggested effects. One of the most studied oils is oregano, with described biological activities reaching well beyond anti-microbial properties; for review, see Leyva-Lopez et al. (2017). This review reports several possible biological effects, suggesting strong potential. On the other hand, it presents oils from 18 different species of oregano, often with completely different results. In addition, this article also warns about reports on adverse effects resulting from the use of these oils.

The differences in activities described in literature might be based on strong effects of drying methods on thyme essential oil composition. In addition, the composition differs widely based on area of harvesting and on thyme species used. It is clear, therefore, that the potential biological effects will widely differ not only among essential oils isolated from different plants or herbs, but also among oils derived from the same plant. This makes it almost impossible to repeat the effects described in the scientific literature or to expect the same results using essential oils from different manufacturers or even from batch to batch.

In an animal model, essential oil supplementation helped alleviate intestinal injury by improving intestinal integrity and modulating immune responses in *Clostridium perfrigens* infected chicken.

In addition to direct effects, a large body of literature has been published on the effects of odors (which is the base of potential effects of essential oils) on the human brain. Several studies focused on mood, alertness, and mental stress. Others focused on task performance or reaction time changes. Most of these studies have shown that individual odors can produce specific effects on human neuropsychological functions. Most of these studies, however, lack in-depth neurophysiological studies on the nature of olfaction and its link to the limbic system. In general, they do not even cite research that shows these links. The idea that essential oils produce effects on the body that are greater than the sum of the individual chemical components of the scents is still popular, but without any significant proof. Psychology and biochemistry communities usually contest these assertions.

Essential oils represent highly questionable parts of biologically active components. Despite reported positive actions on some healthy issues, we do not know anything about the potentially active molecules nor about the possible mechanisms.

References

Al-Tamini, M., Rastal, B., Abu-Reidah, I.M.: Chemical composition, cytotoxic, apoptotic and antioxidant activities of main commercial essential oils in Palestine: A comparative study. Medicines, 3, 2016, doi:10.3390/medicines3040027.

Andrade, M.A., Braga, M.A., Souza Cesar, P.H., Trento, M.V.C., Esposito, M.A., Silva, L.F., Marcussi, S.: Anticancer properties of essential oils: An overview. Curr. Cancer Drug Targets, 18, 2018, doi:10.2174/1568009618666180102105843.

Bhalla, Y., Gupta, V.K., Jaitak, V.: Anticancer activity of essential oils: a review. J. Sci.　　Food Agric., 93: 3643-3653, 2013.

Blowman K., Magalhaes, M., Lemos, M.F.L., Vabral, C., Pires, I.M.: Anticancer properties of essential oild and other natural products. Evidence-Based Complement. Alternat. Med., 2018, doi:10.1155/2-18/3149362.

Curtis, S. *Essential Oils*. Aurum Press, London, 1996.

Farhath, S., Vijaya, P.P., Vimal, M.: Immunomodulatory activity of geranial, geranial acetate, gingerol, and eugenol essential oils: evidence for humoral and cell-mediated responses. Avicenna J. Phytomed., 3: 224-230, 2013.

Leyva-Lopez, N., Gutierrez-Grijalva, E.P., Vazquez-Olivo, G., Heredia, J.B.: Essential oils of oregano: Biological activity beyond their antimicrobial properties. Molecules 22, 2017, doi:10.3390/molecules22060989.

Lu, M., Dai, T., Murray, C.K., Wu, M.X.: Bactericidal property of Oregano oil against multidrug-resistant clinical isolates. Frontiers Microbiol., 9, 2018, doi:10.3389/fmicr.2018.02329.

Orchard, A., van Vuuren, S.: Commercial essential oils as potential antimicrobials to treat skin diseases. Evidence-Based Complement. Alter. Med., 2017, doi:10.1153/2017/4517971

Perez-Roses, R., Risco, E., Vila, R., Penalver, P., Canigueral, S.: Effects of some essential oils on phagocytosis and complement system activity. J. Agricult. Food Chem., 63: 14496-14504, 2015.

Saleh, M.A., Clark, S., Woodard, B., Deolu-Sobogun, S.A.: Antioxidant and free radical scavenging activities of essential oils. Ethnicity Dis., 20: S1-78-S1-82, 2010.

Sharifi-Rad, M., Varoni, E.M., Iriti, M., Martorell, M., Setzer, W.N., del Mar Contreras, M., Salehi, B., Soltani-Nejad, A., Rajabi, S., Tajbakhsh, M., Sharifi-Rad, J.: Carvacrol and human health: A comprehensive review. Phytotherapy Res., 2018, doi:10.1002/ptr.6103.

Sitarek, P., Rijo, P., Garcia, C., Skala, E., Kalemba, D., Bialas, A.J., Szemraj, J., Pytel, D., Toma, M., Wysokinska, H., Sliwinski, T.: Antibacterial, anti-inflammatory, antioxidant, and antiproliferative properties of essential oils from hairy and normal roots of *Leonurus sibiricus* L. and their chemical composition. Oxid. Med. Cell Longevity, 2017, doi:10.1155/2017/7384061.

Tangeveld, W.T., Veldhuizen, E.J.A., Burt, S.A.: Synergy between essential oil components and antibiotics: a review. Crit. Rev. Microbiol., 40: 76-94, 2014.

Vetvicka V, Vetvickova J: bβ,3-Glucan: Silver bullet or hot air? Open Glycosci., 3: 1-6, 2010.

Vetvicka, V., Vetvickova, J.: Essential oils from thyme (*Thymus vulgaris*): Chemical composition and biological effects in mouse model. J. Med. Food, 19: 1180-1187, 2016.

Villarini M, Pagiotti R, Dominici L, Fatigoni C, Vannini S, Levorato S, Moretti M: Investigation of the cytotoxic, genotoxic, and apoptosis-inducting effects of estragole isolated from fennel (*Foeniculum vulgare*). J. Nat. Prod., 77: 773-8, 2014.

9

GINSENG

Ginseng, meaning "man-root", is a slow-growing root herb used medicinally for more than 3000 years by practitioners of traditional Chinese medicine, where it is known as the "king of herbs." It even has its own scientific journal fully dedicated to studies of its effects. The Greek word "panax" means "cure-all", suggesting a long-held notion about its medicinal effects. Traditional use considers ginseng to be a "general tonic."

Several species are commonly referred to as ginseng (Figure 8). The three most commonly used are Asian or Korean ginseng (*Panax ginseng*), American ginseng (*Panax quinquefolius)*, and Siberian (or Russian) ginseng, more properly called "eleuthero" (*Eleutherococcud senticosus*). Although the last one is not in the same genus, it is supposed to have the same effects. In addition, a desert ginseng or Rou Cong Rong (*Cistanche deserticola and C. tubulosa*) with some neuropharmacological effects exists (Gu et al., 2016). Again, this one is not related to the common ginseng.

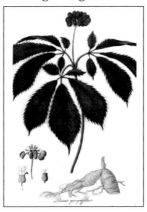

Figure 8   Ginseng

The commercially available formula is usually extracted from the roots, but extracts from stems and leaves are common. To further confuse the situation, the terms "red" and "white" ginseng are often used. "White" means naturally dried ginseng, whereas "red" ginseng is made by steaming and drying fresh root.

Siberian ginseng has been reported to prevent numerous diseases including hepatitis, hyperglycemia, inflammation, and leishmania. Its effects were shown as anti-bacterial, anti-inflammatory, anti-oxidant, and anti-cancer.

The main active components of ginseng are glycosidal saponins known as ginsenosides. There are more than 150 different ginsenosides (saponins) extracts from root, stem, and leaves. For full description of molecules found in ginseng, see Amico et al. (2013). Experiments using mouse and chicken models found that saponins isolated from stems and leaves are the molecules responsible for the adjuvant activities, offering the possibility to change the unpopular aluminum with a natural molecule. Isolated dammarane triterpenes were found to enhance cellular immunity, but each showed a different degree of activity (Tran et al., 2014). A recent study using isolated ginseng saponins emulsified in soybean oil found that they strongly promoted immune response to foot-and-mouth disease vaccine via strong recruitment of neutrophils and macrophages at the injection site, and increased levels of various cytokines, driving the antigen-presenting cells to actively participate in the onset of immunity. Similarly, isolated and standardized saponins enhanced immune response of chickens to oral vaccination against infectious disease.

When tested as possible immunomodulators, studies found stimulation of phagocytosis and increased secretion of inflammatory mediators. Oral administration of ginseng increased activity of natural killer (NK) cells and served as an adjuvant in increasing antibody formation. In addition, reduction of anti-inflammatory cytokines and resulting anti-inflammatory effects has been reported. Readers interested in an excellent review summarizing potential immunostimulating effects of ginseng should read the article Kang et al. (2012). Isolated ginsenoside Rg1 improved survival in a case of polymicrobial sepsis by suppressing the inflammatory response (Zou et al., 2013).

More attention has been focused on ginseng-derived polysaccharides. Published studies showed that these polysaccharides have anti-bacterial, anti-oxidant, anti-inflammatory, and immune-regulatory effects. Some attention has also focused on anti-tumor and chemoprotective effects. Ginseng polysaccharides were found to improve the effects of common anticancer drugs, cyclophosphamide and 5-fluorouracil, and to potentiate the production and release of some mediators of cancer growth and differentiation. The latest biochemical observations showed that the molecules responsible for immune-enhancing effects are, in fact, various glucans (Li et al., 2019).

Some studies have suggested that ginseng has the capacity to reduce stress damage after exercise, probably via reduction of creatine kinase formation. A review of controlled trials found that the performance–enhancing effects of ginseng are not supported by the available evidence. The conflicting results are further confused by significant differences in content of active molecules, as some studies found that ginsenoside content per capsule can vary by more than 20-fold among commercial material.

Relatively few clinical studies have focused on the possible immunomodulatory effects. An interesting study, which followed 227 volunteers treated with influenza vaccine plus placebo or ginseng extract, showed significant reduction of the frequency of colds in groups supplemented with ginseng; this was followed by an increase of antibody titers and NK cell activity (Scaglione et al., 1996). Improved NK cell functions can also be responsible for observed improvements in mice with leukemia. The most interesting part of these experiments was the finding of preventive function, as none of the leukemia-prone mice fed with ginseng developed leukemia (Durairaj and Miller, 2013). Although extensive literature documenting biological effects in laboratory animals exists, results from human studies are conflicting and variable (WHO, 1999). Anti-viral effects were later shown to protect against vaginal herpes simplex virus infection. These effects are probably mediated via increased production of interferon gamma and activation of NK cells.

Using a model of systemic lupus erythematosus, ginsenosides isolated from ginseng roots inhibited B lymphocyte role in the immune regulation, which is normally involved in the development of this disease. As each of the individual samples affected different parts of B lymphocyte activity, it might potentially offer a new treatment option for systemic lupus erythematosus.

Ginseng is also often combined with other natural molecules. For example, delisheng consist of ginseng, mylabris, radix astragali, and venenum bufonis. Its antitumor actions are numerous and strong (gaining a new drug certificate in China), but the multicomponent status makes any conclusions about which substance is responsible for the biological action impossible. A toxicokinetic study of Shenmai, which is a combination of ginseng and *Ophiopagon japonicas*, showed that one month of treatment lowered innate immunity (Yu et al., 2014).

Asian ginseng was found to induce CYP3A4, which could result in decrease of effectiveness of many drugs including chemotherapy and HIV agents, statins, antidepressant, and calcium channel blockers. As such, it is recommended to not take it together with any medication (Malati et al., 2012). Studies on warfarin's effects yielded mixed results, so no recommendation is possible. In addition, ginseng should not be used with estrogens or corticosteroids because of possible additive effects. Further, relatively serious adverse effects, ranging from insomnia, diarrhea, vaginal bleeding, and severe headache, have been described (Ernst, 2002). About 133 reports of human adverse effects were published (Haller et al., 2002). Some case reports showed potentially serious interactions when ginseng was taken with phenelzine (anti-depressant) and imatinib (anti-cancer drug).

American ginseng, although similar to its Asian counterpart, has a different profile of ginsenosides. Therefore, generalization about Asian ginseng should not be extended to American ginseng. However, close monitoring is recommended when taken together with warfarin (Yuan at al., 2004), as it reduces warfarin's effects. Another possible problem might be the attenuation of the postprandial glycemic response, leading to a caution that this supplement should be taken with a meal to prevent unintended hypoglycemia in nondiabetic persons.

Ginseng is also known to affect various aspects of neurodevelopmental and neurological disorders, particularly stroke. The action most probably results from anti-inflammatory effects, but the disagreement exists regarding the effects on cardiovascular parameters. Some studies have found that supplementation with 4 g/day resulted in no effects; other studies found improvements after 1.35 g/day. The summary of current knowledge of ginseng effect in stroke is given by Rastogi et al. (2015). Similarly, studies have found no ergogenic/performance benefits despite testing a variety of exercise constructs.

Like with all herbs or plants with bioactive effects, the

foremost issue is the high amount of individual ingredients present in ginseng extract. The individual extracts will differ in composition based on part of the plant, whether conditions, time of the harvest or geographical location. Some studies only vaguely talk about oligoprotein or polysaccharides, without giving precise information. With over 150 ginsenosides present, even detailed information about one might not be enough. Most studies, if they bother with isolation at all, just describe on percentage of 5-10 individual ginsenosides and briefly mention the presence of additional ones. It is clear that this type of information does not really help to understand the mechanisms of action. In addition, the majority of *in vitro* actions were attributed to the presence of lipopolysaccharide found in bacterial contaminations (Pugh et al., 2008). Another problem connected with ginseng use in humans is its rather high dose, with an active dose recommended to be around 50 g/day.

From the data summarized above, it is clear that even after decades of intensive research, we are not any closer to answering the basic questions about the bioactive molecules in the extracts, mechanisms of action, or the cells affected by ginseng. The bigger problem, however, is that the risks far outweigh the potential benefits of using ginseng as a dietary supplement.

References

Amico, A.P., Terlizzi, A., Damiani, S., Ranieri, M., Megna, M., Fiore, P.: Immunopharmacology of the main supplements: A review. Endocrine Metabolic Immune Disorders – Drug Targets, 13: 283-288, 2013.

Durairaj, P., Miller, S.C.: Neoplasm prevention and immuno-enhancement mediated by daily consumption of a proprietary extract from North American ginseng by elderly mice of cancer-prone strain. Phytotherap. Res., 27: 1339-1344, 2013.

Ernst, E.: The risk-benefit profile of commonly used herbal therapies: Ginkgo, St. John Wort, Ginseng, Echinacea, Saw Palmetto, and Kava. Ann. Intern. Med., 136: 42-53, 2002.

Gum C., Yang, X., Huang, L.: *Cristanches Herba*: A neuro-pharmacology review. Frontiers Pharmacol., 7, 2016, doi:10.3389/phar.2016.00289.

Haller, C.A., Anderson, I.B., Kim S.Y., Blanc, P.D.: An evaluation of selected herbal reference texts and comparison to published reports of adverse herbal events. Adv. Drug. React. Toxicol. Rev., 21: 143-150, 2002.

Kang, S., Min, H.: Ginseng the "immunity boost": The effects of *Panax ginseng* on immune system. J. Ginseng Res., 36: 354-368, 2012.

Li, B., Zhang, N., Feng, Q., Li, H., Wang, D., Ma, L., Liu, S., Chen, C.B., Wu, W., Jiao, L.: The core structure characterization and of ginseng neutral polysaccharide with the immune-enhancing activity. Int. J. Biol. Macromol., 123: 713-722, 2019.

Malati, C.Y., Robertson, S.M., Hunt. J.D., Chairez, C., Alfaro, R.M., Kovacs, J.A., Penzak, S.R.: Influence of *Panax ginseng* on cytochrome P450 (CYP)3A and P-glycoprotein (P-gp) activity in healthy participants. J. Clin. Pharmacol., 52: 932-939, 2012.

Pugh, N.D., Tamta, H., Belachandran, P., Wu, X., Howell, J., Dayan, F.E., Pasco, D.S.: The majority of *in vitro* macrophage activation exhibited by extracts of some immune enhancing botanicals is due to bacterial lipoproteins and lipopolysaccharides. Int. Immunopharmacol., 8: 1023-1032, 2008.

Rastogi, V., Santiago-Moreno, J., Dore, S.: Ginseng: a promising neuroprotective strategy in stroke. Front. Cell. Neurosci., 8, 2015, doi:10.3389/fncel.2014.00457.

Scaglione, F., Cattaneo, G., Alessandria, M., Congo, R.: Efficacy and safety of the standardized Ginseng extract G115 of potentiating vaccination against the influenza syndrome and protection against the common cold. Drug Exper. Clin. Res., 22: 65-72, 1996.

Tran, T.L., Kim, Y.R., Yang, J.L., Oh, D.R., Dao, T.T., Oh, W.K.: Dammarane triterpenes from the leaves of *Panax ginseng* enhance cellular immunity. Bioorg. Med. Chem., 22: 499-504, 2014.

World Health Organization Monographs on Selected Medicinal Plants, Vol. 1, WHO, Geneva, 1999.

Yu, J., Xin, Y.F., Gu, L.Q., Gao, H.Y., Xia, L.J., You Z.Q., Xie, F., Ma, Z.F., Xuan, Y.X.: One-month toxicokinetic study of SHENMAI injection in rats. J. Ethnopharmacol., 154: 391-399, 2014.

Yuan, C.S., Wei, G., Dey, L., Karrison, T., Nahlik, L., Maleckar, S., Kasza, K., Ang-Lee, M., Moss, J.: Brief communication: American ginseng reduces warfarin's effect in healthy patients: a randomized, controlled trial. Ann. Intern. Med., 14: 23-27, 2004.

Zou, Y., Tao, T., Tian, Y., Zhu, J., Cao, L., Deng, X., Li, J.: Gingenoside Rg1 improves survival in a murine model of polymicrobial sepsis by suppressing the inflammatory response and apoptosis of lymphocytes. J. Surg. Res., 183: 260-266, 2013.

10

CURCUMIN

Turmeric, a bright yellow spice isolated from the rhizomes of *Curcuma longa*, is used in traditional Indian cooking (Figure 9). Turmeric/curcumin has a long history as a spice, dye and remedy. In addition to culinary appeal, turmeric and its active ingredient, curcuminoids, have long been used in Indian and Chinese medicine. The medicinal use of turmeric was indicated in Sushruta Samhita, one of the three fundamental texts of Indian traditional medicine, Ayurveda. Besides the ancient literature, the first scientific report related to use of curcumin was published in 1748 (Loeber and Buechner, 1748).

The yellow color of turmeric is due to pigments curcuminoids, with the major factor being curcumin. Curcumin usually is a mixture of three curcuminoids (curcumin, demethocycurcumin, bisdemethoxycurcumin) and volatile oil. Curcumin contains approximately 3-5% of curcuminoids and up to 5% of essential oils and resins (Argawal and Mishra, 2010), varying on geographical region and isolation (for review see Esatbeyoglu et al., 2012). The presence of about 238 compounds has been identified in turmeric, including 109 sesquiterpenes, 68 monoterpenes and 32 diarylheptanoids. The major pharmacologically important compounds are curcuminoids. For details on isolation and composition, see (Bandyopadhyay, 2014).

Numerous studies reported that curcumin has a wide range of biological activities including antimicrobial, antioxidant, antitumor (Ruby et al., 1995) and anti-inflammatory effects. Curcumin was also evaluated in rheumatoid arthritis (Deodhar et al., 1980), inflammatory bowel disease (Bundy et al., 2004) and psoriasis (Heng et al., 2000). In addition, curcumin has some immunosuppressive activities (Gao et al., 2004) including expression of cytokines such as

IL-1 and TNF-α (Chan, 1995, Moon et al., 2004). On the other hand, curcumin enhanced phagocytic activity of macrophages (Bisht et al., 2009). In addition, this report contradicted the effects on cytokines, as production of both IL-1 and TNF-α were increased.

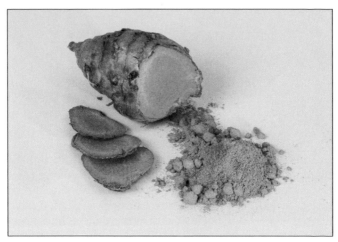

Figure 9 Turmeric

By downregulating transcription factor NF*k*B, curcumin is affecting downstream genes such as myc-v, Bcl-2, COX-2 and MMP9 and subsequently possess cancer-inhibiting properties. In addition, curcumin was reported to improve effects of some chemotherapeutic agents such as doxorubicin. For the list of signaling pathways involved in curcumin-related modulation of cancer growth, see (Bose et al., 2015). Numerous cellular targets include signaling proteins, cytokines, enzymes, adhesion molecules and cell cycle proteins (Shezad et al., 2013).

The differences in the observed effects of curcumin might be caused by differences in bioavailability and metabolism. Some versions of curcumin, particularly nanocurcumin, showed significantly improved efficacy and anti-cancer activity (Basniwal et al., 2014). In an animal model, curcumin was found to improve the therapeutic effects of vaccine in correlation with improved T cell responses in blood of a triple-negative breast cancer model (Singh et al., 2013).

Inflammation is one of the most important processes defending the integrity of organisms against insults. In general, inflammation is a process by which the body's (and substances they produce) protect us from infection with foreign organisms, such as bacteria and viruses. However, in some diseases, the immune system triggers an inflammatory response when there are no foreign invaders to fight off. Acute inflammation is short-lived, chronic inflammation is lasting for weeks. Curcumin has been shown to suppress inflammation in some diseases and promote immune response to acute inflammation (for review see Hamidpour et al., 2015). Early research suggests that curcumin may help with certain conditions, such as osteoarthritis and rheumatoid arthritis, but more research is needed on these benefits.

In breast cancer, curcumin induces apoptosis via p53-dependent Bax induction (Choundhuri et al., 2002). The prevention of tumor invasion and metastasis in a number of animal models, including models of lung, bone, liver, breast, colon, stomach and esophageal cancer, is summarized in (Bandyopadhyay, 2014). In cancer studies, curcumin was found to be particularly effective as a preventive agent against chemotherapy-induced health problems. Gastrointestinal problems and toxicity is one of the most common side effects caused by chemotherapy (and irradiation). Curcumin supplementation improved the intestinal conditions and resulted in chemotherapy-induced weight loss and mucosal atrophy (Yao et al., 2013). In addition, curcumin was found to reduce chemotherapy-induced cardiotoxicity (Venkatesan, 1998), hepatotoxicity (Fetoni et al., 2014) and nephrotoxicity (Zhou et al., 2011). Important observation also found that curcumin targets the process used by tumor cells to escape immune surveillance. Curcumin mediates processes such as restoration of CD4$^+$ and CD8$^+$ populations, reversal of type-2 cytokine bias, reduction of Treg cell populations and suppression of T lymphocyte apoptosis (Bose et al., 2015).

Curcumin supplementation also offered some neuroprotection, again via its anti-oxidant and anti-inflammatory activities (Dikman et al., 2017). Effects on Parkinson's and Alzheimer's diseases are particularly interesting, manifested through maintaining homeostasis of the inflammatory system and facilitation of the heat shock system (for review see Xu et al., 2018). For a detailed analysis of similar effects of curcumin, see (Liu et al., 2018, Xu et al., 2018).

A mouse study showed that orally given curcumin caused significant inhibition of gastric inflammation induced by *Helicobacter pylori* infection (Santos et al., 2015). The aim of our study was to directly compare the antibacterial effects of several different types of curcumin to see if these effects are dependent on the individual type of curcumin. In this study, we used samples with already well-established anti-inflammatory effects. The levels of LPO, an oxidative damage index, were decreased by supplementation with curcumin, and in some cases, almost reached the levels found in non-infected animals. These results suggested that curcumin treatment inhibited the *H. pylori*–induced increase in LPO abundance in the gastric mucosa and that curcumin does have anti-oxidant effects. The next phase of our study focused directly on bacteria and their action. Enumeration of bacterial cells in the infected animal stomach showed that curcumin supplementation reduced the total amount of *H. pylori* bacteria. Next, then analyzed the effects of curcumin supplementation on formation of anti–*H. pylori* IgG antibodies. The results showed the same samples, which reduced the number of bacteria, also increased the formation of specific antibodies. This supports the hypothesis that curcumin has immunostimulating properties and might be developed into potential treatment against *H. pylori* infection (Vetvicka et al., 2016).

In our own study, we investigated the effect of oral supplementation with curcumin on production of cytokines such as IL-4, IL-10, IFN-γ, and TNF-α both *in vitro* and *in vivo*. Mice supplemented with curcumin showed significant protection against LPS-induced endotoxemia effects and against CCL_4-induced hepatotoxicity. In addition, we directly compared the biological effects of several different types of curcumin, showing that only some of them have significant biological activity (Vetvicka and Vetvickova, 2016). The other group also found that curcumin can offer hepatoprotection against various liver injuries induced by drugs, alcohol or pollutants (Xu et al., 2018).

Most of the benefits are attributed to its anti-oxidant and anti-inflammatory activity, thus the best effects are usually found in the management of inflammatory conditions such as arthritis, an exercise-mediated inflammation. For a recent review of the curcumin's effects on human health, see (Hewlings and Kalman, 2017).

Potentially clinically relevant information showed that curcumin (including several derivatives) can inhibit entry of all hepatitis C virus genotypes into human liver cells (Anggakusuma et al., 2014) without having direct anti-viral effects. This mechanism is most probably mediated via effects on membrane fluidity and subsequent impairment of virus binding and fusion. Another suggested use is treatment of atherosclerosis, but again, this hypothesis was supported by one study only (Ouyang et al., 2019).

Despite positive effects mentioned above, a major criticism

of curcumin is its poor bioavailability. In fact, some experts have suggested that given its unstable and nonbioavailable nature, further clinical trials are unwarranted (Nelson et al., 2017). Major reasons for the instability are due to: 1) poor absorption 2) chemical instability 3) fast metabolism 4) rapid elimination. The majority (over 90 percent) of orally given curcumin is excreted in the feces. Serious efforts were devoted to increase its bioavailability, usually with only partial effects. Among others, curcumin is mixed with adjuvants, or as liposomal curcumin, curcumin nanoparticles, curcumin phospholipid complexes or as structural analogs. The best action was found when curcumin was mixed with piperine, the major active component of black pepper. Some studies suggested that curcumin's potential as a therapeutic agent may not solely rely on its bioavailability, but rather its medicinal benefits might arise from its positive effects on the health and function of the gastrointestinal tract; particularly on intestinal microbiota, gut inflammation and oxidative stress (Lopresti, 2018).

As a component of turmeric, curcumin may interact with prescription drugs and dietary supplements. In high amounts, it may be unsafe for women during pregnancy. It may cause side effects, such as nausea, diarrhea, hives or dizziness.

It is not recommended to use curcumin if you have gallstones or a bile duct obstruction. In addition, taking curcumin might slow blood clotting. This might increase the risk of bruising and bleeding in people with bleeding disorders. Curcumin might decrease blood sugar in people with diabetes. Two preliminary clinical studies in cancer patients consuming high doses of curcumin (up to 8 grams per day for 3–4 months) showed no toxicity, though some subjects reported mild nausea or diarrhea (Hsu and Cheng, 2007). On the other hand, several studies found no direct toxicity in patients supplemented with 8 g/day of curcumin for 3 months (Liu et al., 2012). Curcumin intervention on prediabetic individuals can significantly lower the risk of developing type 2 diabetes (Chuengsamarn et al., 2012). However, inhibitory effects of curcumin on drug transporting proteins subsequently increased levels of transporting substrates (Liu et al., 2018). Therefore, curcumin can change pharmacokinetic profiles of the enzymes and increase plasma levels of some drugs. Another warning came from the study which found significant decrease of tamoxifen and endoxifen pharmacokinetics in patients supplementing their treatment with curcumin. These effects can drop the level of active drug below the threshold for treatment efficacy (Hussarts et al., 2019).

For evaluation of clinical trials on curcumin's effects on

humans, see (Xu et al., 2018). Even as some studies are not the highest scientific quality, they still show benefits of curcumin. Clearly, more large trials with controlled placebos are needed to clarify and verify therapeutic effects of curcumin.

Scientific enthusiasm was somehow reduced by Dr. Aggarwal's research fraud. He was forced to retract 19 of his papers describing anti-cancer properties of various herbs and spices, particularly curcumin.

To conclude, curcumin is a cheap and commonly available natural material with solid medicinal effects. The problems are: 1) poor absorption 2) distribution 3) metabolism 4) excretion of curcumin. The bioavailability is low because of poor absorption, rapid elimination and low target organ concentration. Novel formulation and improved routes of administration should help to achieve the optimal therapeutic effects. At present, before the optimal version of curcumin or its derivate is achieved and confirmed. It is, however, rather difficult to recommend most of the currently available curcumins.

References

Anggakusuma, A., Colpitts, C.C., Schang, L.M., Rachmawati, H., Pfaender, F.A., Behrendt, P., Brown, R.J., Bakwitz, D., Steinmann, J., Ott, M., Meuleman, P., Rice, C.M., Plos, A., Pietscham, T., Steinmann, E.: Turmeric curcumin inhibits entry of all hepatitis C virus genotypes into human liver cells. Gut, 63: 1137-1149, 2014.

Argawal, D.K., Mishra, P.K.: Curcumin and its analogues: potential anticancer agents. Med. Res. Rev., 30: 818-823, 2010.

Bandyopadhyay, D.: Farmer to pharmacist: curcumin as an anti-invasive and antimetastatic agent for the treatment of cancer. Front. Chem., 2, 2014, doi:10.3389/fchem.2014.00113.

Basniwal, R.K., Khosla, R., Jain, N.: Improving the anticancer activity of curcumin using nanocurcumin dispersion in water. Nutr. Canc., 66: 1015-1022, 2014.

Bisht, K., Choi, W.H., Park, S.Y., Chung, M.K., Koh, W.S.: Curcumin enhances non-inflammatory phagocytic activity of RAW264.7 cells. Biochem. Biophys. Res. Comm., 329: 632-636, 2009.

Bose, S., Panda, A.K., Murkherjee, S., Sa, G.: Curcumin and tumor immune-editing: resurrecting the immune system. Cell Div., 10, 2015, doi:10.1186/s13008-015-0012-z.

Chan, M.M.: Inhibition of tumor necrosis factor by curcumin, a phytochemical. Biochem. Pharmacol., 49: 1551-1556,1995.

Choudhuri, T., Pal, S., Agwarwal, M.L., Das, T., Sa, G.: Curcumin induces apoptosis in human breast cancer cells through p53-dependent Bax induction. FEBS Lett., 512: 334-340, 2002.

Chuengsamarn, S., Rattanamongkolgul, S., Leuchapudiporn, R., Phisalaphong, C., Jirawatnotai, S.: Curcumin extract for prevention of type 2 diabetes. Diabeti Care, 35: 2121-2127, 2012.

Deodhar, S,D., Sethi, R., Srimal, R.C.: Preliminary study on antirheumatic activity of irritable bowel syndrome symptomology in otherwise healthy adults: a pilot study. J. Alternat. Complement. Med., 10: 1015-1018, 1980.

Dikmen, M., Kaya-Tilki, E., Engur, S., Ozturk, Y.: Neuritogenic activity of epigallocatechin gallate and curcumin combination on rat adrenal pheochromocytoma cells. Fresenius Environ. Bull., 26: 4726-4733, 2017.

Fetoni, A.R., Eramo, S.I., Paciello, F., Rolesi, R., Podda, M.V., Troiani, D., Palludeti, G.: *Curcuma longa* (curcumin) decreases *in vivo* cisplatin-induced ototoxicity through heme oxygenase-1 induction. Otol. Neurotol., 35: e169-177, 2014.

Esatbeyoglu, T., Huebbe, P., Ernst, I.M.A., Chin, D., Wagner, A.E., Rimbach, G.: Curcumin – from molecule to biological function. Angewandte Rev., 51: 2-27, 2012.

Gao, X., Kuo, J., Jiang, H., Deeb, D., Liu, Y., Divine, G., Chapman, R.A., Dulchavsky, S.A., Gautam, S.C.: Immunomodulatory activity of curcumin: suppression of lymphocyte proliferation, development of cell-mediated cytotoxicity, and cytokine production *in vitro*. Biochem. Pharmacol., 68: 51-61, 2004.

Hamidpour, R., Hamidpour, S., Hamidpour, M., Sohraby, M., Hamidpour, R.: Turmeric (*Curcuma longa*): from a variety of traditional medicinal application to its novel roles as active antioxidant, anti-inflammatory, anti-cancer, and anti-diabetes. Int. J. Pharmacol. Phytochem. Ethnomed., 1: 37-45, 2015.

Heng, M.C., Song, M.K., Harker, J., Heng, M.K.: Drug-induced suppression of phosphorylase kinase activity correlates with resolution of psoriasis as assessed by clinical, histological and immunohistochemical parameters. Br. J, Dermatol., 143: 937-949, 2000.

Hewlings, S.J., Kalman, D.S.: Curcumin: A review of its' effects on human health. Foods, 6, 2017, doi:10.3390/foods6100092.

Hsu, CH., Cheng, A.L. Clinical studies with curcumin. Adv. Exp. Med. Biol., 595: 471–80, 2007.

Hussarts, K.G.A.M., Hurkmans, D.P., Oomen-de Hoop, E., van Harten, L.J., Berghuis, S., van Alphen, R.J., Spierings, L.E.A., van Rossum-Schornagel, Q.C., Vastbinder, M.B., van Schaik, R.H.N., van Gelder, T., Jager, A., van Leeuwen, R.W.F., Mathijssen, R.H.J.: Impact of curcumin (with or without Piperine) on the pharmacokinetics of Tamoxifen. Cancers, 11, 2019, doi:10.3390/cancers11030403.

Liu, Z., Huang, P., Law, S., Tian, H., Leung, W., Xu, C.: Preventive effect of curcumin against chemotherapy-induced side-effects. Front. Pharmacol., 9, 2018, doi:10.3389/fpharm.2018.01374.

Liu, A.C., Zhao, L.X., Xing, J., Liu, T., Du, F.Y., Lou, H.X.: Pretreatment with curcumin enhances plasma concentrations of losartan and its metabolite EXP3174 in rats. Biol. Pharm. Bull., 35:145-150, 2012.

Loeber, C.C., Buechner, A.R.: Dissertatio inauguralis medica de curcuma officinarum ejusque genuinis virtutibus. Diss. Inaug. Halae, eds.Praes. A.E. Buchnero, (Halle: Halae Margeburgicae), p.28, 1748.

Lopresti, A.L.: The problem of curcumin and its bioavailability: Could its gastrointestinal influence contribute to its overall health-enhancing effects? Adv. Nutr. 9: 41-50, 2018.

Moon, D.O., Jin, C.Y., Lee, J.D., Choi, Y.H., Ahn, S.C., Lee, C.M., Jeong, S.C., Park, Y.M., Kim, G.Y.: Curcumin decreases binding of Shiga-like toxin-1B on human intestinal epithelial cell line HT29 stimulated with TNF-α and IL1 beta: suppression of p38, JNK and NF-kappaB p65 as potential targets. Biol. Pharm. Bull., 29: 1470-1475, 2006.

Nelson, K.M., Dahlin, J.I., Bisson, J., Graham, J., Pauli, G.F.,

Walters, M.A.: The essential medical chemistry of curcumin. J. Med. Chem., 60: 1620-1637, 2017.

Ouyang, S., Yao, Y.H., Zhang, Z.M., Liu, J.S., Xiang, H.: Curcumin inhibits hypoxia inducible factor-1-a-induced inflammation and apoptosis in macrophages through an ERK dependent pathway. Eur. Rev. Med. Pharmacol. Sci., 23: 1816-1825, 2019.

Ruby, A.J., Kutta, G., Babu, K.D., Rajasekharan, R.N., Kuttan, R.: Anti-tumour and antioxidant activity of natural curcuminoids. Cancer Lett 94: 79-83, 1995.

Santos, A.M., Lopes, T., Oleastro, M., Gato, I.V., Floch, P., Benejat, L., Chaves, P., Pereira, T., Seixas, E., Machado, J., Guerreiro, A.S.: Curcumin inhibits gastric inflammation induced by Helicobacter pylori infection in a mouse model. Nutrients, 7: 306-320, 2015.

Shezad, A., Rehman, G., Lee, Y.S.: Curcumin in inflammatory diseases. Biofactors, 39: 69-77, 2013.

Singh, M., Ramos, I., Asafu-Adjei, D., Quispe-Tintata, W., Chandra, D., Jahangir, A., Zang, X., Aggarwal, B.B., Gravekamp, C.: Curcumin improves the therapeutic effects of Listeria-Mage-b vaccine in correlation with improved T cell responses in blood of a triple-negative breast cancer model 4T1. Cancer Med., 2: 571-582, 2013.

Venkatesan, N.: Curcumin attenuation of acute adriamycin myocardial toxicity in rats. Br. J. Pharmacol., 124: 425-427, 1998.

Vetvicka, V, Vetvickova, J., Fernandez-Botran, R.: Effects of curcumin on Helicobacter pylori infection. Ann. Transl. Med., 4, 2016, doi:10.21037/atm.2016.12.52.

Vetvicka, V., Vetvickova, J.: Strong anti-inflammatory effects of curcumin. J. Nutr. Health Sci., 3, 2016, doi:10.15744/2393-9060.3.205.

Yao, Q., Ye, X., Wang, L., Gu, J., Fu, T., Wang, Y., Wang, Y., Wang, X., Jin, H.C., Guo, Y.: Protective effect of curcumin on chemotherapy-induced intestinal dysfunction. Int. J. Clin. Exp. Pathol., 6: 2342-2349, 2013.

Xu, X.Y., Meng, X., Li, S., Gan, R.Y., Li, Y., Li, H.B.: Bioactivity, health benefits, and related molecular mechanisms of curcumin: Current progress, challenges and perspectives. Nutrients, 10, 2018, doi:10.3390/nu10101553.

11

CINNAMON

Cinnamon is a common spice used in different cultures around the world and is a mainstay of most kitchens. It is extracted from the inner bark of trees from the genus *Cinnamomum* (Figures 10, 11). The name is derived from a Greek word that means sweet wood. In addition to its culinary uses, cinnamon regarded as a remedy for digestive, respiratory and gynecological problems.

There are many types of cinnamon, however there are two varieties that one can most likely find commercially available. The most commonly used source is called Ceylon cinnamon (*Cinnamomum zeylanicum,* sometimes also called *C. verum*), also called "true cinnamon". The oils from this tree contain eugenol, linalool and trans-cinnamaldehyde, which represent over 80% of the total composition. The second source is *Cinnamomum aromaticum (sometimes C. cassia)*. The second one is cheaper, more commonly available and is generally what you will be given at a restaurant or store.

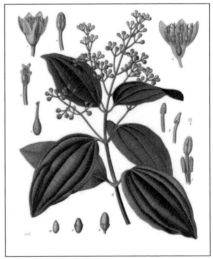

Figure 10 Cinnamon

The main difference between these two cinnamons is the presence of coumarin. The levels of coumarin in Ceylon cinnamon tree is very high and can be hazardous if consumed in high doses for a long time. One teaspoon contains around 5.8 to 12.1 mg of coumarin (German Federal Institute for Risk Assessment), whereas the recommended dose is below 0.1 mg/kg of body weight (Amraham et al., 2010) and the maximum level is set at 2 mg/kg. The high levels of coumarin led some agencies to advocate against the regular use of cassia cinnamon as a supplement in diabetes (European Food Safety Association, 2008).

In addition to the bark, leaves, fruits, flowers and roots of this tree are also supposed to have medical effects. When the volatile oils from individual parts of the tree were directly compared, they significantly differed in chemical composition, meaning they also have different activities. The primary constituents of oils are cinnamaldehyde, eugenol and camphor, with cinnamaldehyde being responsible for the health-related effects. The essential oils of the cinnamon bark can contain up to 80% of cinnamaldehyde.

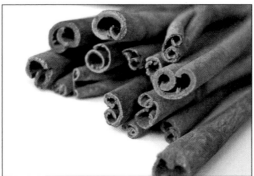

Figure 11   Cinnamon

Some studies have found that cinnamon might help balance blood sugar in those with type 2 diabetes by increasing glucose uptake and by improving insulin sensitivity in tissues. In a clinical setup, people with type 2 diabetes were supplemented with different doses of cinnamon for 40 days. The results demonstrated that all three doses (1, 3, or 6 g per day) reduced the fasting serum glucose, triglycerides, LDL cholesterol and total cholesterol levels (Khan et al., 2003). These effects lasted for 20 more days after the individuals stopped consuming cinnamon. The only problem with this study is the lack of using normal, healthy people. Among suggested health benefits are anti-oxidation via increased production of main anti-oxidant glutathione.

Additional studies found anti-inflammatory and immuno-stimulatory effects. The anti-inflammatory action is mediated by inhibition of production of inflammatory cytokines such as IL-6, IL-1β, and TNF-α and increase of production of anti-inflammatory cytokine IL-10. So far, strong anti-microbial, anti-fungal and anti-parasitic infections were observed under *in vitro* conditions only.

A systematic review of possible medicinal properties of cinnamon from *C. zyelanicum* showed that while this cinnamon can have various health benefits (particularly on hepatotoxicity and during coagulation), data on humans is sparse. Randomized clinical trials are necessary before cinnamon can be recommended (Ranasinghe et al., 2013). Most of the trials used short duration and were poorly designed.

A review of experimental evidence and clinical trials of cinnamon effects on improving glycemic targets in both animal and human models found that cinnamon has potential to be a useful addition to therapy and managing type 2 diabetes. Regardless, the current evidence is still inconclusive and long-term trials are needed (Madagama, 2015). The positive effects on glycemic control were seen both in patients where cinnamon represented the sole therapy and in patients where cinnamon supplemented traditional treatment. However, a 2012 systematic review of 10 randomized controlled clinical trials in patients with type 1 or type 2 diabetes suggested that cinnamon supplementation does not help to reduce glucose levels or glycosylated hemoglobin A1c (Leach and Kumar, 2012).

A phase I clinical trial using only 28 subjects found a decrease of blood pressure and significant reduction of LDL levels without any negative side effects, even after 3 months of supplementation (Ranasinghe et al., 2017).

Animal studies found no significant liver toxicity, but some problems with renal functions (Al-Logmani and Zari, 2009). A detailed study of isolated cinnamaldehyde found significant immunosuppressive effects manifested via inhibition of cell proliferation and induction of apoptosis in immune cells (Roth-Walter et al., 2014). These effects result in the anti-inflammatory properties as it blocks activation of nuclear factor-kB. Moderate doses might be beneficial for healthy organisms, but high doses might be used only in hematopoietic types of cancer. The authors further warned that cinnamaldehyde and cinnamon should not be used in most cancer patients, as this compound might inhibit immune cell activation and/ or directly suppress immune reactions.

References

Abraham K, Wohrlin F, Lindtner O, Heinemeyer G, Lampen A.: Toxicology and risk assessment of coumarin: focus on human data. Mol. Nutr. Food Res., 54: 228-239, 2010.

European Food Safety Association: Coumarin in flavouring and other food ingredients with flavouring properties. EFSA J., 793: 1-15, 2008.

Al-Logmani AS, Zari TA: Effects of *Nigella sativa* L. and *Cinnamomum zeylanicum* Blume oils on some physiological parameters in streptozotocin-induced diabetic rats. Bol. Latinoam. Caribe Plantas, 186: 86-96, 2009.

Khan, A., Safdar, M., Ali Khan, M.M., Khattak, K.N., Anderson, R.A.: Cinnamon improves glucose and lipids of people with type 2 diabetes. Diabetes Care, 26: 3215-3218, 2003.

Leach, M.J., Kumar, S.: Cinnamon for diabetes mellitus. Cochrane Database of Systematic Reviews, 9: CD007170, 2012.

Ranasinghe P, Pigera S, Premakumara GAS, Galappaththy P, Constantine GR, Katulanda P.: Medicinal properties of "true" cinnamon (*Cinnamomum zeylanicum*): a systematic review. BMC Complement. Alt. Med., 13, 2013, doi:1472-6882/13/275.

Ranasinghe P, Jayawardena R, Pigera S, Wathuraptha WS, Weeratunga HD, Premakumara GAS, Katulunda P, Constantine GR, Galappaththy P.: Evaluation of pharmacodynamic properties and safety of *Cinnamomum zeylanicum* (Ceylon cinnamon) in healthy adults: a phase I clinical trial. BMC Complement. Alt. Med., 17, 2017, doi:10.1186/s12906-017-2067-7.

Roth-Walter, F., Moskovskich, A., Gomez-Casado, C., Diaz-Perales, A., Oida, K., Singer, J., Kinaciyan, T., Fuchs, H.C., Jensen-Jarolim, E.: Immune suppressive effect of cinnamaldehyde due to inhibition of proliferation and induction of apoptosis in immune cells: Implications in cancer. PLoS One, 9: e108402,2014.

Madagama AB: The glyceamic outcome of cinnamon, a review of the experimental evidence and clinical trials. Nutrit. J., 24, 2015, doi:10.1186/s12937-015-0098-9.

12

PROBIOTICS

Tremendous changes in lifestyle and eating habits are causing significant and often irreversible changes leading to manifold multiplication of various health problems. There has been, roughly since World War II, an apparent decrease in the prevalence of traditional infectious diseases, with the concomitant increase in immune-related disorders, such as irritable bowel disease, type 1 diabetes and various allergic diseases. One reason might be the reduction of exposure to microbes, which subsequently resulted in an undereducated immune system. In addition, the rise in food products composed of highly refined ingredients has led to decreased consumption of micronutrients, which might be relevant to immune maturation. Dietary strategies might hold promise for immune modulation as well as for maintaining immune homeostasis in the healthy population. The question "which food components impact the functions of the immune system" is simple – all do. Protein malnutrition affects all parts of the immune system. The concept of dietary components being of paramount importance to immune functions is also tangible in the formulation of immunonutritional food. Pro- and prebiotics represent typical products with demonstrated immunomodulatory claims. A number of beneficial health-related effects have been claimed for the pro/pre-biotic category, including effects against antibiotic-associated or traveler's diarrhea, improved stools, as well as wide array of immunity-related health claims.

Proactive action is therefore widely used. Functional foods are often defined as foods that contains some health-promoting components. Sometimes we can find them as: 1) designer food 2) medicinal food 3) nutraceuticals 4) therapeutic food. Within this type of food, probiotics are a small but rapidly expanding area. More than 100 years ago, the idea of probiotics was promoted by a Russian scientist Ilja Metchnikoff, who later won the Nobel Price. Metchnikoff linked health and longevity to ingestion of bacteria present in yogurt. Numerous dietary factors are critical for the evolvement of the microbiome in the large intestine. Several recent studies have shown that numerous diseases are triggered by changes in bacterial communities in the gut. However, this relation is bi-directional, as some types of bacteria in the gut will actually be beneficial. The gut is not just a simple barrier preventing the invasion of bacteria, but is actively involved in the maintenance of a rich and healthy community of gut bacteria. Gastrointestinal problems often develop after receiving heavy doses of antibiotics, because the gut bacteria are affected. A meta-analysis found that probiotics reduced antibiotic-associated diarrhea by 42 percent (Hempel et al., 2012). Similarly, a review article found that certain strains of probiotics, particularly Bifidobacteria, can help with constipation (Dimidi et al., 2014).

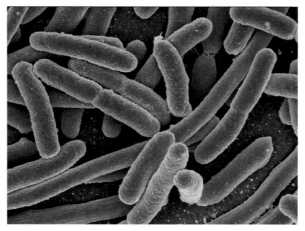

Figure 12   Probiotic bacteria

Prebiotics are non-digestible food ingredients that help to stimulate the growth and activity of bacteria in the digestive system. The whole idea was introduced in 1995 by Gibson and Roberfroid (1995). The second term, sometimes mixed with the term "prebiotics," is probiotics. It might be of interest that the term "probiotic" was initially used as an antonym of the term "antibiotics" and its translation from Greek means "for life." Probiotic refers to viable microorganisms that promote or support a beneficial balance of the autochthonous microbial population of the gastrointestinal tract. These are live microorganisms that are beneficial to the organism. It is important to remember that these bacteria are nonpathogenic microorganisms. A number of genera of bacteria and yeast are used as probiotics, including 1) *Lactobacillus* 2) *Leuconostoc* 3) *Pediococcus* 4) *Bifidobacterium* 5)

Saccharomyces 6) *Enterococcus*. The most common probiotics are lactic acid bacteria (*Lactobacillus acidophilus*) and bifidobacteria (*Bifidobacterium lactis*). These bacteria are usually consumed as part of fermented food with added live cultures. The use of yogurt is the most common example. It is important to note the conditions in most food are not optimal for long-term survival of bacteria. Therefore, we have to remember that the presence of bacteria mentioned on the label does not necessarily reflect reality. The nutraceutical potential and bioactive properties of polysaccharides including glucan have been investigated in depth during the last decade. For detailed information, see a comprehensive review by Sharma and Devi (2014). Probiotics can reduce 1) diarrheal incidence 2) lactose intolerance 3) lower serum cholesterol 4) stimulate immunity 5) control infections 6) can maintain a healthy intestinal balance protecting against colon and bladder cancer.

In general, probiotics are live microorganisms that, when delivered in sufficient amounts, confer health benefits on the host. Probiotics are a big and rapidly growing business and are now among the most popular supplements. The number of organisms in a daily dose can range from 1 billion to more than 250 billion. Many manufacturers boast that their products contain unique probiotics or a unique combination of strains that make them even better, and often charge a premium price.

Given the well-established health effects of glucan, it is not surprising that a combination of glucan with probiotics was studied. Using a fish model, a recent study demonstrated strong synergy in stimulation of immune system between glucan and probiotic strain *Shewanella putrefaciens* (Guzman-Villanuev et al., 2014).The direct studies of the probiotic effects of glucans produced by lactic acid bacteria showed that these polysaccharides are not only a safe food additive, but also have unique properties that might facilitate its application in the food industry as a viscosifying and gelling agent. A detailed study testing prebiotic activity of glucans with nine probiotic strains of *Lactobacillus, Bifidobacterium* and *Enterococcus* shows strong prebiotic activities, strongly dependent on types of glucan and strain specificity (Synytsya et al., 2009).Our own experiments used LactoSpore. LactoSpores are *Bacillus coagulans* in the form of spores able to withstand the acidic environment of the stomach and to start to proliferate within the gastrointestinal tract. We found that probiotics alone had only a limited effect on some immune and physiological reactions. When combined with cinnulin (special version of cinnamon), it offered significant improvements in blood glucose levels and improved survival rates in mice with experimental colitis (Vetvicka and Vetvickova, 2013). It is important to note that cinnulin alone had almost no activity at all.

Food enhanced with barley-derived glucans significantly enhanced probiotic performance of beneficial bacteria. The main reasons for these effects are that they are highly fermentable by intestinal microbiota and enhance growth rate and lactic acid production of microbes in the human intestine. In addition, glucans have positive effects on bacterial adhesion to enterocyte cells (Arena et al., 2014).

It is particularly important to remember the numbers game. The human gastrointestinal system contains approximately 39 trillion bacteria, most of which reside in the large intestine. The majority of these bacteria are beneficial; they crowd out their harmful cosins, break down fibrous material and produce some vitamins such as vitamin B12 and vitamin K. The science behind the pick of the best probiotic strains is still not adequate and manufacturers often select the specific bacterial strains because they know how to grow them, not because they are best adapted to the conditions in the human intestine. In addition, the viability of bacteria in food is decreasing with their storage. The numbers are showing another problem – with many trillions of bacteria in the intestine, a few hundred billion bacteria in a yogurt serving is usually not enough to change the diversity of microbiome.

Probiotics are considered safe overall for healthy people, with short-term side effects that may include mild bloating or gas formation. In general, probiotics are a promising field of research and may one day be used therapeutically. However, there is not enough solid evidence to recommend their widespread use. Closer look at the science behind various claims shows that most of the health claims for probiotics are hype, as the majority of studies have failed to reveal any benefits in individuals who are already healthy. The bacterial supplementation seems to help only those suffering from a few specific intestinal disorders. Vague claims that various probiotics support healthy gastrointestinal or digestive system are meaningless. Larger and longer studies are needed to test particular bacterial strains for specific conditions.

References

Arena, M.P., Caggianiello, G., Fiocco, D., Russo, P., Torelli, M., Spano, G., Capozzi, V.: Barley β-glucan-containing food enhances probiotic performance of beneficial bacteria. Int. J. Mol. Sci., 15: 3025-3039, 2014.

Dimidi, E., Christodoulides, S., Fragkos, K.C., Scott, S.M., Whelan, K.: The effect of probiotics on functional constipation in adults: a systematic review and meta-analysis of randomized controlled trials. Am. J. Clin. Nutr., 100: 1075-1084, 2014.

Gibson, G. R., Roberfroid, M. B.: Dietary modulation of the human colonic microbiota: introducing the concept of prebiotics. J. Nutr., 125: 1401-1412, 1995.

Guzman-Villanuev, A.T., Tovar-Ramirez, D., Gisbert, E., Cordero, H., Guardiola, F.A., Cuesta, A., Meseguer, J., Ascencio-Valle, F., Esteban, M.A.: Dietary administration of β-1,3/1,6-glucan and probiotic strain Shewanella putrefaciens, single or combined, on gilthead seabream growth, immune responses and gene expression. Fish Shellfish Immunol., 39: 34-41, 2014.

Hempel, S., Newberrym S.J., Maher, A.R., Wang, Z., Miles, J.N.V., Shanman, R., Johnsen, B., Shekelle, P.G.: Probiotics for the prevention and treatment of antibiotic-associated diarrhea: systematic review and meta-analysis. JAMA, 307: 1959-1869, 2012.

Sharma, M., Devi, M.: Probiotics: A comprehensive approach toward health foods. Crit. Rev. Food Sci. Nutr., 54: 537-552, 2014.

Synytsya, A., Mickova, K., Synytsya, A., Jablonsky, I., Spevacek, J., Erban, V., Kovarikova, E., Copikova, J.: Glucans from fruit bodies of cultivated mushrooms Pleurotus ostreatus and Pleurotus eryngii: structure and potential prebiotic activity. Carbohydrate Polym., 76: 548-556, 2009.

Vetvicka, V., Vetvickova, J.: Physiological effects of a combination of cinnulin with probiotics. Am. J. Immunol., 9: 103-109, 2013.

13

Transfer Factor

The term "transfer factor/s" has various unrelated meanings in science. One was developed by Lawrence, originated from human cells and consisted entirely of amino acids. A second use of the term transfer factor applies to a likely different entity derived from cow colostrum or chicken egg yolk. These are marketed as an oral dietary supplement under the same name citing claims of benefit to the immune system. Generally, transfer factor is a chemical material taken from either humans or animals with already established immunity against certain diseases.

The idea originated in Chase's observation that cells taken from the peritoneum of guinea pigs that had been immunized could transfer immunity when injected into guinea pigs that had never been exposed to the antigen. Subsequent research attempted to uncover how the cells imparted their effects. Later, Henry Sherwood Lawrence discovered that partial immunity could be transferred even when the immune cells had undergone lysis. This indicates that cells did not need to be fully intact in order to produce immune effects (Lawrence, 1955). His later studies showed that only the factors less than 8000 Daltons were required to transfer this immunity; he named these to be "transfer factors". In Lawrence's work, transfer factor referred to "an extract of human white blood cells that could transfer a type of immunity called cell-mediated immunity", and was never isolated from bovine colostrum. The real transfer factor is sometimes called Lawrence Transfer Factor, to make sure it corresponds to the original invention. The original definition defined this material as dialyzable leukocyte extract that can transfer antigen-specific immunity from a person whom tests positive for the antigen in a delayed hypersensitivity skin test manner to a person negative for the same antigen. Transfer factor is a small molecule, and it has been the center of a scientific mystery, in part because Dr. Lawrence and other scientists were unable to identify it precisely. Some scientists suspect that transfer factor represents bits of many molecules. At present, neither the precise chemical nature, nor the exact molecular mechanisms of action have been defined. However, transfer factors have been shown to provide both therapeutic and prophylactic benefits.

While Dr. Lawrence's colleagues recognized the importance of his discovery, his science went largely unreported. In the early 1940s, only a few years before discovery of transfer factor, antibiotics were introduced and pharmacology gained new prominence as the frontline for battling disease. For years, his observation was ignored, until 1970 when the use of transfer factor started in primary immunodeficiencies (Levin et al, 1970). Since then, transfer factor has been evaluated in numerous clinical trials (Fudenberg and Pizza, 1993).

Another setback occurred in the 1980s with the first blood screening tests for HIV infection and the fear of contracting HIV through blood-born products. Additional problems were caused by the scandal from two researchers at Harvard working with transfer factor, who noted that "original positive results may not have been obtained by the procedures described". Culmination of these events set back the interests of research community for decades. Subsequently it took decades before serious research in transfer factor started again (Wang et al., 2017).

Serum-derived transfer factor improved the ability of recipient animals to survive lethal infection with canine parvovirus or salmonellosis via changes in cytokine production (Willeford et al., 2017). Similar results were found in case of: 1) tuberculosis 2) leprosy 3) viral challenges 4) *varicella* infection 5) leishmaniosis 6) toxoplasmosis. An experimental model of pulmonary tuberculosis showed that both human and mouse transfer factor restored the expression of some cytokines provoking inhibition of bacterial proliferation and resulting in increase of survival. In addition, mouse transfer factor in combination with chemotherapy has synergistic effects producing faster elimination of lung bacteria (Fabre et al., 2004).

The history of cellular-derived transfer factor as a treatment effectively ended in the early 1980s. While the research world was initially excited by the possibility that a small molecule could affect the immune system, the concept of small molecules having such profound biologic effect had not been proven. Despite several successes in using transfer factor to treat human disease and uncover immune effects, one then-prominent researcher was exposed for falsifying data related to his work on transfer factor and guinea pigs. This effectively cast all of transfer factor science in a negative light (Ched, 1974). This scandal was followed shortly thereafter by the discovery of the interleukin-1 and thus attention further shifted towards research on interleukins. By 1973, it was discovered that blood products could harbor viruses such as hepatitis A, indicating that transfer factor treatments derived from human or cow blood cells had the potential to transmit these diseases. With the eventual discovery of HIV/AIDS as an additional blood-borne disease, most researchers viewed a product derived from blood as an unsafe treatment since screening for hepatitis B and HIV/AIDS would not be developed until much later.

Most recently, transfer factor has been harvested from sources other than blood, and administered orally, as opposed to intravenously. This use of transfer factors from sources other than blood has not been accompanied by the same concerns associated with blood-borne diseases, since no blood is involved. Transfer factor-based nutritional supplements have become extremely popular throughout the world. However, the way transfer factor works is still not clear.

Colostrum is a form of milk produced by the mammary glands of mammals in late pregnancy. Colostrum also contains multiple immune modulating molecules, including antibodies. Based on studies noting an overlap in the observed *in vitro* effects between a molecule contained in colostrum called colostrinin and the dialyzable leukocyte extract, a hypothesis formed that the two were the same. There has been no recent research investigations comparing the two entities and thus there is no verifiable evidence that either colostrum or egg whites do or do not contain the cellular product that shares the name transfer factor. The orally available transfer factor is not obtained from humans or from blood products of any mammal or animal and does not carry the presumed risks of contracting blood borne or animal tissue derived diseases. The problem is that all science was done on specific transfer factor. It is true that few studies found positive effects of colostrum-derived transfer factor, but it was obtained from previously immunized cows against specific antigens. This type of material was able to transfer the immunity from cows to chickens (Wilson et al., 1988). Similarly, it transferred the immunity to young calves (Radosevich et al., 1985). In all cases, the transfer factor and the subsequent transfer of immunity was specific (Krishnaveni, 2013).

For a long time transfer factor was used only by injection, most of all by subcutaneous injection. However, some studies using mouse models showed that there are no substantial differences in response to either oral or injected transfer factor (Kirkpatrick et al., 1995). No similar study in humans exists, except one study using one patient only (Jones et al., 1981). It is clear that a one-patient-study has no real value.

Colostrum/egg-derived transfer factors have been promoted as treatment for a large number of diseases and health concerns, but have not been proven effective in the treatment of any of these conditions. The United States Food and Drug Administration regulates transfer factors as dietary supplements, the FDA issued a warning notice to a website selling transfer factors that they have not been proven to be effective or safe in the treatment of any condition, nor have there been any biological licenses or new drug applications produced for the substance.

Most of clinical studies of transfer factors have been based on the specificity of each transfer factor, e.g., transfer factor that is specific for *Herpes* infection will prevent recurrent infection with this virus, but not with anything else. However, the companies marketing most of current transfer factor use a different approach - they ignore the specificity and make nonspecific claims of boosting immune system.

From the safety point of view, transfer factor from human sources is considered to be possibly safe when used up to 2 years, whereas transfer factor derived from cows is considered possibly safe when used up to 3 months. Mad cow disease has not been transmitted by transfer factor.

Despite the deep skepticism for its use in clinical practice, the use of transfer factor as tailor-made immunotherapy in the treatment of some diseases is quite valuable. But before its administration, it is important to evaluate the specificity, potency, and the best dose, to individualize the treatment for each patient. To do that, however, is beyond its use as a supplement, as transfer factor needs to be specific.

References

Chedd, G.: Transfer factor - Another scandal? New Scientist, 64: 920–921, 1974.

Fabre, R.A., Perez, T.M., Aguilar, L.B., Rangel, M.J., Estrada-Garcia, I., Hernandez-Pando, R., Parra, S.E.: Transfer factor as immunotherapy and supplement of chemotherapy in experimental pulmonary tuberculosis. Clin. Exp. Immunol., 136: 215-223, 2004.

Fudenberg, H.H., Pizza, G.: Transfer factor 1993. New Frontiers. Prog. Drug Res., 42: 309-400, 1993.

Jones, J.F., Schumacher, M.J., Jeter, W.S., Pritchett, R.F., Fulginiti, V.A., Wedgwood, R.J.: Treatment of childhood combined Epstein-Barr virus/cytomegalovirus infection with oral bovine transfer factor. Lancet, 2: 122-124, 1981.

Kirkpatrick, C.H., Hamad, A.R., Morton, L.C.: Murine transfer factors: dose-response relationships and routes of administration. Cell. Immunol., 164: 203-206, 1995.

Krishnaveni, M.: A review on transfer factor an immune modulator. Drug Invent. Today, 5: 153-156, 2013.

Lawrence, H.S.: The transfer in humans of delayed skin sensitivity to streptococcal M substance and to tuberculin with disrupted leucocytes. J. Clin. Investig., 34: 219–130, 1995.

Levin, A.S., Spitler, L.E., Stites, D.P., Fundenberg, H.H.: Wiscott Aldrich syndrome, a genetically determined cellular immunologic deficiency: clinical and laboratory responses to therapy with transfer factor. Proc. Natl. Acad. Sci. USA, 67: 821-828, 1970.

Radosevich, J.K., Scott, G.H., Olson, G.B.: Delayed-type hypersensitivity responses induced by bovine colostral components. Am. J. Vet. Res., 46: 875-878,1985.

Wang, J.F., Park, A.J., Rendini, R.N., Levis, M.D.: Lawrence transfer factor: Transference of specific immune memory by dialyzable leukocyte extract from a CF8+ T cell line. J. Drugs Dermatol., 16: 1198-1206, 2017.

Willeford, B.V., Shapiro-Dunlap, AT., Willeford, K.O.: Serum derived transfer factor stimulates the innate immune system to improve survival trait in high risk pathogen scenarios. Drug Dev. Res., 78: 189-195, 2017.

Wilson, G.B., Poindexter, C., Fort, J.D., Ludden, K.D.: *De novo* initiation of specific cell-mediated immune responsiveness in chicken by transfer factor (specific immunity inducer) obtained from bovine colostrum and milk. Acta Virol., 32: 6-18, 1988.

14

ECHINACEA

The *Echinacea* species used for treatment of respiratory infections are *E. purpurea, E. pallida,* and *E. angustifolia.* These tall and hardy perennial plants are endemic to North America, where they were first used by Native Americans in the Great Plains region and later adopted by white settlers (Figure 13). The first official reports of *Echinacea* were found in Flora Virginica in 1762 and later in the Materia Medica Americana from 1787, recommending it for treating skin problems and respiratory tract infections. Suggestions linking this plant to immunomodulation date back to 1913, way before the birth of immunology as a science. From the 1930s to the 1970s, antibiotic development resulted in a sharp decline in *Echinacea* use, but due to a subsequent disenchantment with the medical establishment, an herbal medicine renaissance in the 1980s led to renewed interest in *Echinacea*'s benefits. Historically, *Echinacea* has been recommended for treatment of syphilis and septic wounds, but also as an antitoxin for snakebites. Its long history is not exactly an argument for efficacy, but it does indicate some degree of safety. The longevity of its use suggests that it is not just an ancient fad, but perhaps has a true benefit. Currently, public interest is growing rapidly and *Echinacea* is the top-selling herbal product in the United States, commanding up to 10% of the herbal market.

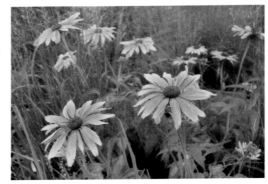

Figure 13 *Echinacea*

During the latter part of the 19th century, and the first 30 years of the 20th century, *Echinacea* was the preferred treatment for infections. All this changed after 1928, when Alexander Fleming discovered penicillin. Various preparations of *Echinacea* are among the most widely used herbal medicines. Numerous studies described its immunostimulative effects, mostly on macrophage activation. Changes in lymphocyte numbers and activities were also reported, but the data is less convincing. So far, the effects seem to be due to multiple components rather than the individual chemical compounds found in extracts. An in vitro study of herb and roots, as well as preparations standardized to phenol acid or echinacoside contents, found that the unstandardized material enhanced activities of macrophages, whereas standardized material was immunologically inactive.

Different preparations sold under the common name "*Echinacea*" can show substantial disparities in composition. These variations are primarily due to the different species of *Echinacea* as well as different modes of extraction. In addition, extracts can be prepared from roots, flowers, stalks, whole plants, or any combination of these. There are considerable differences in the constituents of *Echinacea* across the species and their respective parts. The main active molecules involve alkamides, caffeic and ferulic acid esters, essential oils (which are a mixture of many components), polysaccharides, glycoproteins, polyacetylenes, and echinacosides, but no single constituent is considered responsible for the biological effects. Some studies suggested that pharmacology, chemistry and biological properties of caffeic acids derivatives do not contribute to activity (Barnes et al., 2005, Sharifi-Rad et al., 2018). Composition of the root, when compared to other parts, is substantially different with more volatile oils and pyrrolizidine alkaloids. *Echinacea* has a complex mix of active substances, some of which are said to be antimicrobial, while others are believed to have an effect on the human immune system. These constituents all showed high chemical variability, mostly due to several endogenous and exogenous factors including genetic traits, plant organs, climatic factors, drying, extracting and storage conditions, and overall health of the plants.

Respiratory tract infections are the most frequently encountered illnesses in the Western world. These infections involve common cold and influenza, both of which can be manifested by a wide variety of symptoms. Data from the National Institute of Allergy and Infectious Diseases estimate that up to one billion cases of colds are experienced in the Unites States every year with overall costs of 39 billion dollars (Adams et al., 1999).

Due to suggested anti-infectious effects, it has been used for furunculosis and other skin conditions, and numerous upper respiratory tract problems. Lately, *Echinacea*-containing products are exceptionally popular in Germany, with more than 800 products on the market. It is also extremely popular in the United States, commanding up to 10% of the herbal market. Some studies found anti-microbial effects *in vitro,* but the effects are usually caused by stimulation or inhibition of cytokines, not by direct anti-microbial action. For detailed review of potential effects, see Sharifi-Rad et al. (2018).

Evaluations of *Echinacea* effects are dubious, as approximately one-half of the published studies showed no effects at all (Holst et al., 2014). In addition, The National Institutes of Health (NIH) warn consumers to be careful regarding some *Echinacea* products that are on the market, as *Echinacea* products are commonly mislabeled; some have been tested and found to have no *Echinacea* in them at all. The term "standardized" may sound impressive, but has no real meaning. The results of one *Echinacea* species, using extraction method and dosage, cannot be extrapolated to a dissimilar preparation because chemical composition will differ. This is clearly confirmed by the study evaluating chemically characterized fractions from aerial parts on myelopoiesis (Ramasahayam et al., 2011). Although laboratory-made samples were active, commercial extracts showed no activity, probably due to conflicting effects by medium-chain fatty acids presumably derived from a non-plant additive.

Additional comparative studies found some effects on flu-like symptoms and upper respiratory problems (both bacterial and viral), but most of the studies relied on self-reporting, which significantly lowered their quality. Consensus of the comparative studies indicates that when used to prevent the illness, *Echinacea* provides little or no benefits. If consumed at the onset of symptoms, it might have some effects. An additional study suggested that *Echinacea* might be beneficial to those with known immune problems, but showed little effects on a healthy immune system (Melchart et al., 1995). An excellent summary of immunostimulating effects of *Echinacea* is reported by Smejkal and Rjaskova (2016).

Despite its popularity, clinical studies on *Echinacea* have produced mixed results, mostly due to the poor characterization of the extract and the use of different species and/or plant parts. A more precise study using highly purified extract from *E. augustifolia* consisting of complex polysaccharides and phenylethanoid echinacoside, and lacking alkamides, showed promising results in improving immune response to influenza vaccine (Di Pierro et al., 2012). A review of 16 randomized clinical trials also resulted in inconclusive results. A study testing polysaccharide arabinogalactan showed effects on macrophages, but not on B or T lymphocytes.

A systematic review of controlled clinical trials on possible reduction of risk of respiratory tract infections also offered mixed results. On the one hand, most of the described effects showed significant improvements; on the other hand, most of the 26 studies used varying materials, from different monoextracts to preparations containing other ingredients. Some meta-analyses found positive effects particularly for ethanolic extracts (Schapowal et al., 2015). However, the methodological quality of most studies was low and only eight trials reached 50% of maximum possible points (Melchart et al., 1994). A large comparative study reviewed the literature from 1966 to 1999 on the use of *Echinacea* for treatment of the common cold. The results were not conclusive due to numerous flaws of the studies and the use of non-standardized material. The only conclusion reached was that *Echinacea* is safe (Giles et al. 2000).

Recent meta-analysis of numerous clinical trials in children with respiratory tract infection found no effects (Anheyer et al. 2018). The basic difficulties plaguing such studies are flaws in design, small number of patients, and variability in measured outcomes, dosing, and treatment schedule. In addition, *Echinacea* in liquid form has a rather distinct taste, making a genuine blind test virtually impossible.

The importance of standardization was clearly shown with Echinaforce, which is the standardized extract of *Echinacea* manufactured in Switzerland. The use of this extract in a placebo-controlled study showed not only stimulation of immunity, but also direct action against a series of viruses without any side effects (Schapowal, 2013). Similar effects were also found in a meta-analysis of effects in the prevention of induced rhinovirus colds. Additional studies showed possible attenuation of the mucosal immune suppression occurring after intense exercise.

Quality randomized, double-blind studies with valid clinical outcome are a rarity in about more than 400 studies that have detailed *Echinacea* use. The literature reveals conflicting data regarding *Echinacea's* ability to prevent or reduce the severity and duration of various infections. Some studies supported its ability to reduce the severity of symptoms of upper respiratory infections and other bacterial infections (Brinkeborn et al., 1999); however, many others reported no effects (Barrett et al., 2002, Grimm and Muller, 1999, O'Neil et al., 2008). One of these negative studies even found an increased rate of rash in *Echinacea*-supplemented children (Taylor et al., 2003). In a review of 11 published clinical trials on this subject, only 2 met all criteria expected from a good clinical trial (Caruso and Gwaltney, 2005). The results of these two studies were negative; whereas, the results of the studies with lower quality were positive. The authors of the review concluded that the possible therapeutic effectiveness cannot be established. A study performed at the University of Washington included 407 children with a total of 707 upper respiratory problems (Taylor et al., 2003). This double-blind study showed that the use of *Echinacea* failed to affect the duration or severity of cold symptoms in the children. A mild rash appeared in 7% of the treated group, compared to 3% in placebo group. These results mirror a previous study.

Most studies suggest that use of the extract shortens the duration and severity of colds and other upper respiratory problems when given as soon as the symptoms become evident. However, trials of long-term use as a preventative have not shown positive results (Block and Mead, 2003).

Although there is good data resulting from trials testing extracts in the treatment of upper respiratory infections, these trials are limited both in size and methodological quality. Therefore, the effectiveness of *Echinacea* in treatment of illnesses or in enhancing our health has yet to be proved with reasonable certainty. Some comparative studies suggest that *Echinacea* is effective in reducing the duration and severity of some symptoms, but these effects are noted only with certain preparations (Percival, 2000) and differ based on type of extract and the health state of an individual. As the reviews give contradictory results, it is particularly difficult for consumers to interpret, especially as there are gaps between the body of evidence and the diverse summaries. An interesting report provided an illustrative overview of how information from different systematic reviews is summarized on the internet. The authors compared published studies with 12 webpages presenting the results. Only three of webpages used all of the studies, the rest only one or two. In addition, the explanation of results was substantially different, leaving consumers little or no possibility to assimilate the evidence (Hart and Dey, 2009).

Echinacea has no direct anti-bacterial or anti-viral activity. Instead, it is believed to indirectly affect the immune system by activating macrophages. The immunostimulating effects are suggested to be caused by three mechanisms––phagocytosis activation, fibroblast stimulation, and the increase of respiratory activity. There are a few reports suggesting some antibacterial effects, but these are mostly anecdotal and describe the plant used externally on wounds. A high-quality study revealed that immunostimulatory effects are mediated via activation of macrophages and their functions, most of all IL-6 and IL-12 production. Seemingly, *Echinacea* initiates a signaling cascade within macrophages through both TLR4-dependent and -independent mechanisms (Sullivan et al., 2008).

Echinacea extracts have also been traditionally used in wound healing, where the effects are attributed to its polysaccharide fraction by producing a hyaluronic acid–polysaccharide complex.

A direct comparison of an alcohol extract from three widely used *Echinacea* species showed effects on both innate and adaptive immune responses. The effects were dependent on individual species and more pronounced in stress animals, putting the role of *Echinacea* in healthy populations in doubts (Zhai et al., 2007).

Other animal studies showed protection against stress-induced immunosuppression in mice, immunoregulatory effects by reducing Treg cell numbers and function, as well as increased phagocytic activity in dogs.

In vitro antiradical capacity of *Echinacea* extracts has been documented, including scavenging of superoxide anion radicals and decreasing peroxide levels. Therefore, addition of *Echinacea* products to foods seems to be a promising way of introducing natural antioxidant agents.

The most studied forms are the juice from the aerial portions of *E. purpurea* and alcohol extracts from *E. augustifolia* roots. However, it is uncertain which part of the plant, of which species, or in which formulation (squeezed sap, hydro alcoholic extract, dried powder) offers the most evidence for efficacy. This is particularly interesting when we take into consideration a study by Benson et al. (2010), which directly compared the immunological effects of extracts from different parts of the plant. The authors found that whereas root extracts stimulated the expression of various markers and receptors, leaf extracts inhibited it. Similarly, IL-6 and TNF-α secretion was stimulated by root extract, but unchanged by leaf extract, suggesting that extracts from leaves with additional ability to inhibit enzymatic activity of COX-2 and antigen presentation, have more immunosuppressive than immunostimulatory action. There are conflicting results about effects on CYPIA1 and CYP3A4, so caution should be taken when *Echinacea* is combined with medications that are metabolized by these CYP enzymes, including anti-psychotic and anti-depressant medications (Gorski et al., 2004).

A gene-based study compared the biological effects of root and stem plus leaf extracts and found opposite effects; i.e., one extract had enhancing effects and the other had inhibitory effects (Wang et al., 2006). These results seem to have clinical potential, because if we could really attach individual effects to an exact component, we might obtain tools for tailor-made modification of the immune system. However, these data stress the potential danger of using crude extracts full of biologically active substances that often act against each other.

Stimulators of immune reactions are usually not recommended for use in various autoimmune diseases, mostly due to the general understanding that these diseases are caused by an aberrant immune system. Dietary consumption of *Echinacea* in mice with diabetes, type I, resulted in strong increase of NK cell numbers. As these cells are often considered instrumental in modulating and ameliorating diabetes, the authors hypothesize about a possible new approach to the treatment of this disease. However, the study did not find any improvements by *Echinacea* supplementation (Delorme and Miller, 2005).

Potential problems

German Commission E approved oral use of *Echinacea* with suggested time limit of 6 weeks. In addition, the same committee cautioned that *Echinacea* should not be used in systemic diseases such as tuberculosis, leukemia, multiple sclerosis, and autoimmune diseases. The Australian Adverse Drug Reaction Advisory Committee received 11 reports of adverse reactions during one year, including hepatitis, asthma, rash, and anaphylaxis.

Another problem resulting from *Echinacea* supplementation was described recently (Corhssen, 2006). However, only four allergic skin reactions were described during 6-year period. Barrett (2003) reported the potential risk connected with the use of various *Echinacea* extracts. A prospective study of 206 pregnancies in which the fetus was exposed to *Echinacea* found no significant differences in pregnancy outcomes, delivery methods, maternal weight changes, or birth weight. In addition, no animal research has been able to find a calculable lethal dose, and extended dosing of laboratory animals failed to demonstrate adverse reactions on any tested parameters. However, the analytical review of the published studies states that despite the low frequency of adverse effects, such as mild dyspepsia, headache, and dizziness, serious reactions can occur. Caution is advised for patients with a history of hypersensitivity to sunflower seed or ragweed (Giles et al., 2000). In addition, National Registry of Drug-Induced Ocular Side Effects have received several reports of eye irritation and conjunctivitis secondary to topical *Echinacea* use (Fraunfelder, 2004). A detailed study of complementary interventions in asthma, allergy and immunity found risks of hepatotoxicity, exacerbation of allergies and asthma (Bielory, 2004).

Echinacea may also cause hepatotoxicity and should not be used with other known hepatotoxic drugs such as anabolic steroids, methotrexate, and ketoconazole (Budriznski and Foster, 2000). The direct effects are still unknown, as it lacks 1,2-saturated necrine ring associated with hepatotoxicity of alkaloids. A recent review and assessment of medicinal safety data of orally-used *Echinacea* found no significant reasons for possible problems (Ardjomand-Woelkart and Bauer, 2016). Similarly, no *Echinacea* drug interaction has been documented. The metabolic and transport proteins, such as cytochrome P450 enzymes, can be affected and result in changes of drug transport (Shord et al., 2009).

Another problem might be the suppression of the effectivity of oral contraception. *Echinacea* extracts often contain hypericin, which is known for complex increase of elimination of hormonal contraception from blood. This might result in lower effectivity of contraception and unplanned pregnancy.

Research on *Echinacea* is limited, and to a large extent, exists only in Germany. Future research is clearly needed to identify, not only the most effective species of *Echinacea*, but also distinguish between the efficacies of the different plant parts. Although many of the active compounds have been identified, the mechanisms of action, bioavailability, potency, synergistic and side effects are still unknown. Based on the current knowledge, the use of *Echinacea* products does not guarantee any significant positive effects.

References

Adams, P.F., Hendershot, G.E., Marano, M.A.: Current estimates from the National Health Interview Survey 1996. In: *Vital and Health Statistics Series 10*. Data from the National Health Survey, 1999, pp. 1-203.

Anheyer, D., Cramer, H., Lauche, F., Saha, F.J. Dobos, G.: Herbal medicine in children with respiratory tract infection: Systematic review and meta-analysis. Acad. Pediat., 18: 8-19, 2018.

Ardjomand-Woelkart, K., Bauer, R.: Review and assessment of medicinal safety data of orally used Echinacea preparations. Planta Med., 82: 17-31, 2016.

Barnes, J., Anderson, L.A., Gibbons, S., Phillipson, J.D.: *Echinacea* species (*Echinacea angustifolia* (DC.) Hell., *Echinacea pallida* (Nutt.) Nutt., *Echinacea purpurea* (L.) Moench): a review of their chemistry, pharmacology and clinical properties. J. Pharm. Pharmacol., 57: 929-954, 2005.

Barrett, B.: Medical properties of *Echinacea*: A critical review. Phytomedicine, 10: 66-86, 2003.

Barrett, B.P., Brown, R.I., Locken, K., Maberry, R., Bobula, J.A., D'Alessio, D.: Treatment of the common cold with unrefined *Echinacea*. A randomized, double-blind, placebo-controlled trial. Ann. Intern. Med., 137:1-18, 2002.

Benson, J.M., Pokorny, A.J., Rhule, A., Wenner, C.A., Kandhi, V., Cech, N.B., Shepherd, D.M. *Echinacea purpurea* extracts modulate immune dendritic cell fate and function. Food Chem. Toxicol., 48: 1170-1177, 2010.

Bielori, L.: Complementary and alternative interventions in asthma, allergy and immunology. Ann. Allergy Asthma Immunol., 93: S45-S54, 2004.

Block, K.I., Mead, M.N.: Immune system effects of *Echinacea*, ginseng, and Astragalus: A review. Integr. Canc. Therap., 2: 247-267, 2003.

Brinkeborn, R.M., Shah, D.V., Degenring, F.H.: Echinaforce and other *Echinacea* fresh plant preparations in the treatment of the common cold. A randomized placebo controlled, double-blind clinical trial. Phytomedicine 6: 1-6, 1999.

Budzinski, J.,W., Foster, B.C., Vandenhoek, S., Arnason, J.T.: An *in vitro* evaluation of human cytochrome P450 3A4 inhibition of selected commercial herbal extracts and tinctures. Phytomedicine 7: 273-282, 2000.

Caruso, T.J., Gwaltney, J.M.: Treatment of the common cold with *Echinacea*: A structured review. Clin. Inf. Dis., 40: 807-810, 2005.

Cohrssen, A.: *Echinacea's* immune effects – possibilities and pitfalls – two cases. Explore 2: 232-233, 2006.

Delorme, D., Miller, S.C.: Dietary consumption of *Echinacea* by mice afflicted with autoimmune (type I) diabetes Effect of consuming the herb on hemopoietic and immune cell dynamics. Autoimmunity, 38: 453-461, 2005.

Di Pierro, F., Rapacioli, G., Ferrara, AT., Togni, S.: Use of standardized extract from *Echinacea augustifolia* (*Polinacea*) for the prevention of respiratory tract infections. Alt. Med. Rev., 17: 26-41, 2012.

Fraunfelder, F.W.: Ocular side effects from herbal medicines and nutritional supplements. Am. J. Ophthalmol. 138: 639-647, 2004.

Giles, J.T., Palat, C.T., Chien, S.H., Chang, Z.G., Kennedy D.T.: Evaluation of Echinacea for treatment of the common cold. Pharmacotherapy 20: 690-697, 2000.

Gorski, J.C., Huang, S.M., Pinto, A., et al. The effect of *Echinacea* (*Echinacea purpurea* root) on cytochrome P450 activity *in vivo*. Clin. Pharmacol. Ther., 76: 89-100, 2004.

Grimm, W., Muller, H.H.: A randomized controlled trial of the effect of fluid extract of *Echinacea purpurea* on the incidence and severity of colds and respiratory infections. Am. J. Med., 106: 259-260, 1999.

Hart, A., Dey, P.: *Echinacea* for prevention of common cold: An illustrative overview of how information from different systematic reviews is summarized on the internet. Preventive Med., 49: 78-82, 2009.

Holst, L., Havnen, G.C., Nordeng, H.: *Echinacea* and elderberry – should they be used against upper respiratory tract infections during pregnancy? Frontiers Pharmacol., 5, 2014, doi:10.3389/fphar.2014.00031.

Melchart, D., Linde, K., Worku, F., Bauer, R., Wagner, H.: Immunomodulation with *Echinacea* – a systematic review of controlled clinical trials. Phytomedicine 1: 245-254, 1994.

Melchart, D., Linde, K., Worku, F., Sarkady, L., Jolzmann, M., Jurcic, K., Wagner, H.: Results of five randomized studies on the immunomodulatory activity of preparations of *Echinacea*. J. Alt. Comp. Med., 1: 145-160, 1995.

O'Neil, J., Hughes, S., Lourie, A., Zweifer, J.: Effects of *echinacea* on the frequency of upper respiratory tract symptoms: a randomized, double-blind, placebo-controlled trial. Ann. Allergy Asthma Immunol., 100: 384-388, 2008.

Percival, S.S.: Use of *Echinacea* in medicine, Biochem Pharmacol., 60: 155-158, 2000.

Ramasahayam, S., Baraka, H.N., Abdel Bar, F.M., Abuasal, B.S., Widriechner, M.P., El Sayed, K.A., Meyer, S.A.: Effects of chemically characterized fractions from aerial parts of *Echinacea purpurea* and *E. angustifolia* on myelopoiesis in rats. Planta Med., 77: 1883-1889, 2011.

Shapowal, A.: Efficacy and safety of Echinaforce in respiratory tract infections. Wien Med. Wochenschr., 163: 102-105, 2013.

Schapowal, A., Klein, P., Johnston, S.I.: *Echinacea* reduces the risk of recurrent respiratory tract infections and complications: A meta-analysis of randomized controlled trials. Adv. Ther., 32: 187-200, 2015.

Shord, S.S., Shah, K., Lukose, A.: Drug-botanical interaction: A review of the laboratory, animal, and human data for 8 common botanicals. Integrat. Canc. Ther., 8: 208-227, 2009.

Shrifi-Rad, M., Mnayer, D., Morals-Braga, M.F.B., Pereira Carneiro, J.N., Bezerra, C.F., Coutinho, H.D.M., Salehi, B., Martorell, M., del Mar Contreras, M., Soltani-Nejad, A., Uribe, Y.A.H., Yousaf, Z., Iriti, M., Sharifi-Rad, J.: *Echinacea* plants as antioxidant and antibacterial agents: From traditional medicine to biotechnological applications. Phytotherapy Res., 2018, doi:10.1002/ptr.6101.

Smejkal, K., Rjaskova, V.: Use of plant extracts as an efficient alternative therapy of respiratory tract infections. Cas. Slov. Farm. 65: 139-160, 2016.

Sullivan, A.M., Laba, J.G., Moore, J.A., Lee, T.D.G.: *Echinacea*-induced macrophage activation. Immunopharmacol. Immunotoxicol., 30: 533-574, 2008.

Taylor, J.A., Weber, W., Standish, L., et al. Efficacy and safety of *Echinacea* in treating upper respiratory tract infections in children. A randomized controlled trial. JAMA 290: 2824-2830, 2003.

Wang, C.Y., Chiao, M.T., Yen, P.J., Huang, W.C., Hou, C.C., Chien, S.C., Yeh, K.C., Yang, W.C., Shyur, L.F., Yang, N.S.: Modulatory effects of *Echinacea purpurea* extracts on human dendritic cells: A cell- and gene-based study. Genomics 88: 801-808, 2006.

Zhai, Z., Liu, Y., Wu, L., Senchina, D.S., Wurtele, E.S., Murphy, P.A., Kohut, M.L., Cunnick, J.E.: Enhancement of innate and adaptive immune functions by multiple *Echinacea* species. J. Med. Food, 10: 423-434, 2007.

15

GLUCAN

Polysaccharides in general and glucans in particular, have a long history as immunomodulators. As early as the beginning of the 18th century, it was known that certain infectious diseases showed a therapeutic effect on malignant processes. The dedicated use of such therapy dates from around the middle of the 19th century, at which time Bush performed experiments in search of curing sarcoma by infecting patients with an acute streptococcus bacterial infection of the dermis. Coley repeated these therapeutic procedures towards the end of the 19th century. However, the early researchers had no knowledge of the molecule responsible for the observed effects.

Much later, the attention was focused on zymosan. Although zymosan was able to stimulate a nonspecific immune response, initially it was not clear what component of this rather crude composition was responsible for the activity. When zymosan was examined in detail, glucan was identified as the component of primary effect. It was subsequently isolated and its immunological effects were investigated.

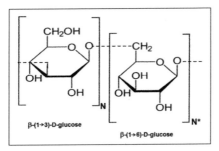

Figure 14 Glucan molecule

Intensive research of immunomodulating activities of β-glucan (hereinafter referred to as glucan) was also conducted in Japan and they arrived at glucan via a different route. In Asian medicine, consuming different medicinal mushrooms (shiitake, maitake, reishi, etc.) has been a long tradition. In detailed studies of the biological effects of these mushrooms, in particular their anticancer action, glucans were again found to be the main cause of nonspecific immunomodulation. This initial investigation was conducted by Goro Chihara at Teikyo University in Kawasaki, who isolated glucan from the shiitake mushroom, which he referred to as lentinan. This glucan, with some subsequent modification, was approved as a drug in 1983 and has been successfully used.

During decades of research, numerous types of glucan have been isolated and described (schematic representation of the basic molecular structure of glucan molecule is shown in Figure 14). In scientific literature, you can find hundreds of different components, all under the name glucan. Unfortunately, not all glucans were created equal and glucans widely differ not only in physicochemical properties, such as branching or molecular weight, but also in biological properties. Some of the described glucans show little activity and others have no biological activities. It is necessary to constantly monitor all conditions during the isolation and purification processes; otherwise, the final product will have limited biological activity, if any. The concentration of effective glucan in a product and the dose bear a strong relationship to immunological effects.

Yeasts are the major source of glucans in Western countries. The Far East (Japan, China, and East Russia) traditionally focuses on mushrooms (based on their folk remedies). A high amount of seaweed existing in western France resulted in a seaweed-derived glucan called "Phycarine" produced by Goemar Laboratories. In addition, numerous glucans isolated from various grains originate from Canada and New Zealand.

Glucans can be isolated from almost every species of yeast, and the reason for the popularity of *Saccharomyces cerevisiae* is purely based on availability. Glucan forms part of the yeast cell wall, together with mannan, proteins, lipids, and small amounts of chitin. Glucans represent a major structural component of the cell wall in fungi and some plants. Different physicochemical parameters, such as solubility, primary structure, molecular weight, branching and polymer charge, all play a role in determining whether the polysaccharide modulates immune reactions. Some conclusions can be made, though. Branched or linear 1,4- glucans have very limited activity, if any. Glucans with 1,6 configuration, usually have limited activity. The highest stimulation of defense reactions has been achieved with glucans that have a 1,3 configuration with additional branching at the position 0-6 of the 1-3 linked D-glucose residues. Among all glucans, those with a 1,3 configuration are best characterized in the literature. An excellent review of glucans as biological response modifiers and the relationship between structure and functional activity is given by Bohn and BeMiller (1995).

The original studies of glucan effects on the immune system focused on mice. Subsequent studies demonstrated that glucan has a strong immunostimulating activity in a wide variety of other species including earthworms, bees, shrimp, fish, chickens, rats, rabbits, guinea pigs, dogs, sheep, pigs, cattle, and humans. Based on these results, it has been concluded that glucans represent a type of immunostimulant that is active over the broadest spectrum of biological species, and that it is one of the first immunostimulants active across the evolutionary spectrum.

The major challenge is to remove the impurities, such as mannoproteins and lipids (attached to the end points of the side branches in the intact cell wall), without the significant loss of desirable biological activity. I am often asked the question: "Can I eat the whole yeast (or mushrooms)? They surely contain glucan." The answer is easy–– whole yeasts alone are not the optimal source of active beta glucan. This is due primarily to their content of available glucan not being high enough, so we would have to consume large quantities of yeast. In addition, our gastrointestinal tract is not prepared to digest whole yeast and to extract pure glucan from yeast cell walls. When glucan is not adequately purified, it will contain numerous impurities, often acting against the biological effects of glucan molecules. Some of these impurities can block the specific binding site on the membrane of immunocytes, further inhibiting the binding. In addition, due to their larger size, they are normally not phagocytized by gut cells and, therefore, insufficient potential glucan can enter our body. The same is true about the glucan "versions" offering mushroom powder instead of purified glucan.

Glucans from fungi, yeast, grain, and seaweed are well-known biologic response modifiers that function as immunostimulants against numerous health problems including infectious diseases and cancer. Unlike most other natural products, properly purified glucans retain their bioactivity. This allows us to characterize how glucans work on a cellular and molecular level.

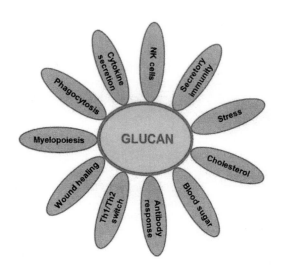

Figure 15 Biological effects of glucan

      Based on the multiple biological effects of glucan (summarized in Figure 15), it is not surprising that this natural immunomodulator is also involved in the fight against cancer. Despite the fact that most tumors are recognized by the immune system, the antibody response is usually not strong enough to kill a cancer growth. Even a completely healthy immune system cannot adequately deal with fast-growing cancer cells. Glucan is extremely important, as it is able to cooperate with antibodies. After the tumor cells have been recognized as foreign, specific antibodies are released and subsequently bind to the cancer cells. Following this binding of antibodies, the C3 fragment of complement coats the surface of cancer cells. The glucan-primed cells, such as macrophages and specifically natural killer (NK) cells and neutrophils, then recognize these antibody-C3 coated cells and kill them. Without glucan, the destruction would not take place and the situation would be compounded very quickly. Figure 16 shows the effect of glucan supplementation on inhibition of cancer.

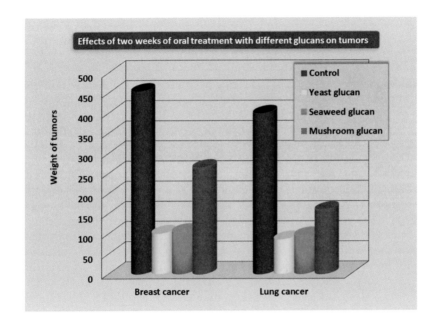

Figure 16

There are multiple positive effects of glucan in tumor therapy. One is the direct stimulation of macrophages and NK cells. Macrophages form the first line of defense and protect our body against any type of invading cells including cancer cells. NK cells represent a special subtype of "bloodthirsty" lymphocytes and have an extremely important function—to specifically recognize and kill tumor cells. Together, these cells form a defensive line that guards the integrity of our body. Their job is not easy and considering they perform this function literally 24/7, it is easy to see how they can become exhausted. Therefore, they can use all the help they can get.

In order to fully investigate the mechanisms and potential utility of glucan in immunotherapy, it was necessary to develop a suitable mouse system. First, mouse leukocyte CR3 was shown to function as a receptor for glucans in the same way as human CR3. Next, it was shown that the primed state of macrophages and NK cells remained detectable for up to 24 hours after a short interaction with glucan (Vetvicka et al., 1997). Monoclonal antibodies are currently being evaluated in an increasing number of disorders including cancer. Although many patients respond to the antibody treatment, remissions are often transient. For example, more than 50% of lymphomas recurrent after rituximab treatment, failed to respond the second time. The reasons for this resistance to the antibody treatment are currently unknown but might include loss of antigen, pharmacokinetic variations among individual patients, or resistance to complement activity. It is clear, however, that for a truly reliable antibody treatment, there is a strong need for a synergetic support.

Numerous recent studies have shown that glucan is extremely active in cooperation with antibodies that naturally occur in cases of cancer (Hong et al., 2003, 2004). We have to keep in mind that antibodies alone cannot make tumor cells disappear. However, following the binding of antibodies on the surface of cancer cells, C3 fragments of complement coat the cancer cells. The glucan-primed cells, such as blood neutrophils, macrophages, and NK cells, then specifically recognize these complement-antibody complexes and kill the tumor cells. Most tumors are recognized by the immune system; however, the antibody response is usually light and often is not strong enough to kill a cancer growth. Here comes glucan to the rescue. The glucan-activated immunocytes recognize and kill cancer cells coated with antibodies. Without the glucan-caused activation of immunocytes, the cancer cells remain coated with antibodies but no killing occurs. It is important to note that similar effects can be also observed with neutrophils.

The studies of glucan's activities were first focused on cancer. In addition to their effect in the treatment of cancer, glucans have been demonstrated to protect against infection with both bacteria and protozoa in several experimental models and were shown to enhance antibiotic efficacy in infections with antibiotic-resistant bacteria. The protective effects of glucans were shown in experimental infection with *Leishmania major, Leishmania donovani, Candida albicans, Toxoplasma gondii, Streptococcus suis, Plasmodium berghei, Staphylococcus aureus, Escherichia coli, Mesocestoides corti, Trypanosoma cruzi, Eimeria vermiformis,* and anthrax (*Bacillus anthracis*).

Some detailed studies have shown significant synergy of glucan with common antibiotics. Original studies done on guinea pigs demonstrated that simultaneous administration of glucan and antibiotics elevated the ability of animals to resist lethal septic infection by antibiotic-resistant bacteria (Kernodle et al., 1998). At the same time, those results suggested that the use of glucan can help to lower the doses of antibiotics in commercial farming, which is particularly important since there is a strong effort to completely abandon the use of antibiotics in all farmed animals. Other study focused on Lyme disease and, from obtained data, we concluded that food supplementation with glucan might offer a new way to suppress the effects of *B. burgdorferi* infection. The exact mechanisms are still unclear, but probably involve stimulation of immune reactions, particularly T_h2-related cytokines.

Besides bacterial infections, glucans were repeatedly shown to positively influence viral infections. Our own study found enhancement of immune response against influenza challenge by oral stimulation with glucans (Vetvicka and Vetvickova, 2015). Glucan also increased survival of cells infected with hepatitis virus strain MHV-A 59 in mice. There are some data from human studies showing positive effects on HIV-infected patients (Itoh et al., 1990).

In the last two decades, extensive research by numerous scientific groups has helped to reveal the extraordinary effects that glucan has on our immune system. Upon binding to specific receptors (CR3, Dectin-1) present on the membrane of cells involved in immune reactions, activation of cells starts. This activation consists of several interconnected processes that include increased chemokinesis, chemotaxis, migration of macrophages to particles to be phagocytosed, degranulation leading to increased expression of adhesive molecules on the macrophage surface, adhesion to the endothelium, and migration of macrophages to tissues. In addition, glucan binding also triggers intracellular processes that are characterized by the respiratory burst after phagocytosis of invading cells such as the formation of reactive oxygen species and free radicals. Glucan binding also begins signaling processes that lead to activation of other phagocytes and secretion of cytokines and other substances initiating inflammation reactions (e.g., interleukins IL-1, IL-9, TNF-α). Basically, the binding of glucan to these receptors tricks the neutrophils and NK cells into thinking that the cancer cells are invading yeast cells (full of glucan) and guides them in their destruction.

Glucans are extremely beneficial to people undergoing chemotherapy. Chemotherapy drugs kill cells indiscriminately. The hope is that they will kill fast-dividing (i.e., cancerous) ones more quickly than healthy ones. However, healthy cells are very much under attack. This is why people become so weak. Their immune system pretty much disappears, whereas taking glucan will protect your immune system cells while allowing the drugs to do their job on the cancerous ones. The production of white blood cells will start again very quickly after your chemotherapy treatment, and you will recuperate more quickly. Studies have also shown increased survival times for patients who took glucans at the same time as chemotherapy. So, to summarize: when people take glucans at the same time as chemotherapy, they have less side-effects, do not feel quite as ill, and the effects of chemotherapy are greatly improved. In other words, the treatment is more likely to work. The effects of glucan here are the same as in the case of irradiation (see Figure 17).

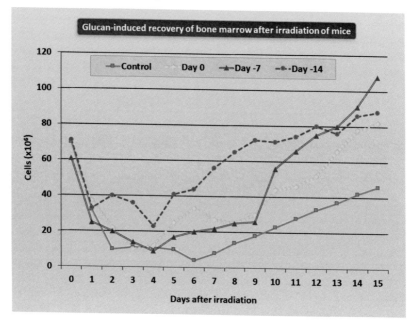

Figure 17

As glucan effects on cancer have been demonstrated in every tested animal or human solid tumor model, it is not surprising that glucan is currently being investigated in more than 90 clinical trials worldwide (Vannucci et al., 2013, Hong et al., 2003, Fujimoto et al., 1991).

The most pronounced effect of glucans consists of augmentation of phagocytosis and proliferative activities of professional phagocytes––granulocytes, monocytes, macrophages, and dendritic cells. In this regard, macrophages, considered to be the basic effector cells in host defense against bacteria, viruses, multicellular parasites, tumor cells, and erroneous clones of our own somatic cells, play the most important role. The miraculous effects of glucan do not end with the activation of immunocytes. In addition to the ability to stimulate the cells of the immune system to perform optimally and maximally, glucan also "cares" about their numbers. It is well established that all cells involved in immune reactions originate from common precursors called stem cells that originate from the bone marrow. The influx of new cells from the bone marrow is steady throughout one's entire life. However, the formation and migration of newly formed cells is limited and, here again, glucan comes to the rescue. It strongly stimulates the production of precursor cells in the bone marrow, resulting in a more rapid flow of new immunocytes into the bloodstream, and subsequently into the various organs throughout the body. These effects are important not only under normal conditions, as the increased amount of immunocytes in circulation means increased surveillance against potential invaders, but particularly in the case of extreme stress, such as in cancer, where the limited influx is further reduced by the exhaustion of the immune system and by treatments such as irradiation and chemotherapy.

Another important role of glucan action involves the effects on the gastrointestinal tract. In inflammatory bowel disease, the application of anti-inflammatory drugs is the first line of pharmaceutical intervention. Given the rapid increase in cases of inflammatory bowel disease, there is a growing need for anti-inflammatory drugs but also for substances able to moderately control inflammation. Efficient biologicals for targeted treatment options are available; however, many of these have side effects and are cost intensive. Ideally, uptake of substances isolated from natural dietary products or even by consumption of specific natural products would provide a great benefit for the compliance and acceptance of such therapeutic approach by the patients and concomitantly lower expenses significantly. We have demonstrated that the oral administration of glucan from *Pleurotus ostreatus* reduced the intestinal inflammation and dextran sulfate sodium–induced symptoms of colitis in mice. Preliminary results showed that this glucan could also potentially prevent colorectal cancer incidence along with inflammatory bowel disease and reduce the expression of the proliferating-associated marker (Vetvicka et al., 2019).

An interesting study used a glucan isolated from *Pleurotus ostreatus* in a model of acute colitis induced by intracolonic administration of acetic acid. Intraperitoneal administration of glucan and luminar pretreatment resulted in a significant reduction of the colonic damage score and colonic wet weight. Four weeks of oral administration reduced the extent of mucosal damage but failed to prevent the increase of myeloperoxidase in the injured colon (Nosalova et al., 2001). Additional effects of glucan were found in a model of irritant-induced gastric lesions. When lesions were induced by application of either HCl or ethanol, gastric ulcerogenic effects of glucan isolated from *Aureobasidium pullulans* were evaluated. The study showed significant effects including suppression of neutrophil infiltration, expression of several inflammatory cytokines, and cell adhesion molecules. In addition, the levels of heat shock protein 70 and mucin were increased. This type of heat shock protein has strong anti-inflammatory activity, most likely via inhibition of the NF-kB activity resulting in lower production of pro-inflammatory cytokines (Chen et al., 2006).

Additional effects of glucan involve cholesterol. The link between elevated cholesterol levels and the risk of coronary disease has been clearly established. In addition, cardiovascular disease related to elevated blood cholesterol levels is still the most common cause of death in humans in western countries. Since none of the current cholesterol-lowering drugs are without side effects, the search for a natural modulator of cholesterol concentrations is an important task. Once again, glucan comes to the rescue. In 1997, the US Food and Drug Administration (FDA) approved the use of the following health claim on food product packages: "A diet high in soluble fiber from whole oats and low in saturated fat and cholesterol may reduce the risk of heart disease." In 2005, barley was included as a source of soluble fiber in this claim. In May 2008, the FDA added certain oat products to a health claim linking soluble fiber and decreased risk of coronary heart disease.

Similarly, in 2006 the European Food Safety Authority gave a positive opinion on the following health claim for food containing glucan: "Regular consumption of glucan can actively lower/reduce blood LDL cholesterol and total cholesterol." It is clear that glucan (most often from oats) can be linked to cholesterol reduction and the science is sufficiently robust to have merited health claims in a range of countries. Indeed, such a claim has existed in Sweden since 2002, the UK since 2004, and France since 2008.

In addition to the effects of glucan oriented towards the immune system, glucans were also shown to reduce the total and LDL cholesterol levels of hypercholesterolemic animals and patients. Nearly 50 years ago, the possible effects of dietary fiber were first suggested by Keys and these effects were later found to be associated with glucans (Tietyen et al., 1990). The cholesterol-lowering effects of fibers are routinely associated with glucans. Due to the high consumption of oats or oat bran, attention has mostly focused on the relationship of oat-derived glucan to cholesterol levels in both animals and humans (Sima et al., 2018). In men, long-term clinical studies using soluble forms of glucans demonstrated decreased blood cholesterol in hypercholesterolemic patients (Braaten et al., 1994). In addition, glucan decreased the atherosclerotic effects, hyperlipemia and hepatic damage of liver, which were induced by means of highfat diet (Wilson et al., 2004).

The effects of glucan on blood sugar are less studied. Older studies suggested that glucans might reduce blood glucose concentrations after eating, possibly by delaying bowel movements so dietary glucose is absorbed more gradually. Some studies have shown the hypoglycemic activity of natural glucans. Additional studies have demonstrated the strong hypoglycemic activity of synthetic polysaccharides. Some follow-up experiments even suggested that small synthetic oligosaccharides lower the blood sugar similar to natural glucans, which would rule out the possible effects via fiber action. However, the mechanisms remain unknown. In our experiments, we focused our attention on the effects of glucan administration on the levels of blood sugar. Feeding with glucan did not significantly affect the sugar levels. However, a different situation was found when we used mice with experimentally-induced hyperglycemia. After two weeks of feeding, Glucan #300 significantly lowered the sugar levels to almost normal. A longer application of glucan resulted in additional significant activity of ImmunoFibre glucan. Full details of experiments describing the effects of glucans on cholesterol and blood sugar are available (Vetvicka and Vetvickova, 2007).

More and more papers describe the healing properties of glucan including changes in arthritis. A study using osteoarthritis induced by anterior cruciate ligament transection and partial meniscectomy revealed that 84 days on continuous oral administration of glucan resulted in a lower degree of articular stiffness and histological cartilage damage. The optimal glucan dose was found to be 42.5 mg/kg (Kim et al., 2012). The exact mechanisms of glucan action on arthritis are unclear; the authors speculate a possible connection with inhibition of bone loss and acceleration of bone formation.

Some recent studies suggested that glucan may play a role in alleviating allergic problems. The mechanisms of the role of glucan in allergies are not, as of yet, fully established. One possible hypothesis is that glucan effects manifest via decreasing pro-inflammatory cytokines such as IL-6 and TNF-α and increasing secretion of IL-10 and accession of cellular antioxidants (Senoglu et al., 2008). Similar results showing improved Th1/Th2 balance were achieved using an OVA-sensitized allergy in mice. Subsequent studies showed that the oral administration of glucan downregulated the specific antibody IgG$_1$ and IgE in asthma-induced animals.

In our research, we focused on children with respiratory problems. Upper respiratory infections have the highest incidence of acute illness in the developed world. According to the estimates, the average adult has three colds per year and the average schoolchild up to 10. Although patients with complications may benefit from antibiotic or inhaler treatment, current medicine has very little to offer for uncomplicated infections. There is no doubt that a need for a safe, effective, inexpensive treatment for chronic respiratory problems exists. Using a long-term cooperation with Sanatorium for Respiratory Disease EDEL, which is located in North Moravia in an area of extremely low air pollution, we conducted a series of clinical, placebo-driven trials of the effects of a 30-day supplementation with Glucan #300 on immune parameters in children with chronic respiratory problems. The sanatorium offers not only optimal therapeutic treatment, but also a complexity of additional treatments, including speleotherapy. As a part of long-term observation, randomly selected groups of children with respiratory problems were treated with 100 mg of orally administered glucan. Several parameters were evaluated at the beginning and at the end of the study. Three parameters—salivary calprotectin, albumin, and C-reactive protein—were used for the evaluation of acute inflammatory response and the quality of the nonspecific immunity of children. Data summarized in Figure 18 show the strong effects of glucan supplementation on all three tested parameters.

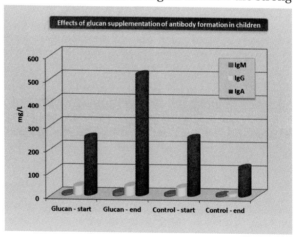

Figure 18

Changes in salivary albumin are an indicator of local immune response to the environmental stress; C-reactive protein is an acute inflammation protein registering inflammatory responses. Pleiotropic function of calprotectin is mostly connected with anti-inflammatory reactions, including antimicrobial mechanisms, where calprotectin acts as a barrier forming antimicrobial shield (Richter et al., 2014 a, b, c).

Glucans unmistakably occupy a prominent position among immunomodulators. They are clearly defined by their origin and structure. In addition, they are relatively inexpensive and possess extremely low risk of negative side effects. In addition to effects in anti-infectious and anti-cancer immunity, novel studies clearly demonstrated significant palliative effects of glucan in allergy, arthritis, gastrointestinal tract diseases, stress reduction, and reduction of cholesterol levels.

Conclusion

Despite the overwhelming number of scientific papers, use of glucans is still restricted because far too many individual glucans have been used that differ widely in source, solubility, molecular weight, branching, and other physicochemical characteristics. With various routes of administration added to the mix, confusion is clear. This data diversity can be only solved by comparative studies, which are still rare (Vetvicka and Vetvickova, 2010, Zhao et al., 2014, Vetvicka and Vetvickova, 2016). The direct conclusion from these studies is clear—no direct connection between source and immunological activities exists. In addition, highly purified and highly active glucans have strong and pleiotropic biological effects; whereas, poorly isolated glucans have only average or minimal biological effects.

Glucans still are, often by nonprofessionals, criticized because of insufficiently defined preparations and unclear or nonspecific effects. Fortunately, in the last 15 years, research in reputable laboratories from all around the world has finally reached the stage where the basic mechanisms of glucan effects are well established and individual activities have been clearly explained. We do believe that glucan will soon hold the position ascribed more than four decades ago. With over 90 clinical trials currently ongoing, the question of whether other countries will follow Japan, where glucan has officially been in use since 1983, is not if, but when.

References

Bohn, J. A., BeMiller, J. N.: (1-3)-β-D-glucans as biological response modifiers: a review of structure-functional activity relationships. Carbohydrate Polymers, 28: 3-14, 1995.

Braaten, J.T., Wood, P.J., Scott, F.W., Wolynetz, M.S., Lowe, M.K., Bradley-White, P., Collins, M.W.: Oat beta-glucan reduces blood cholesterol concentration in hypercholesterolemic subjects. Eur. J. Clin. Nutr., 48: 465-474, 1994.

Chen, H., Wu, Y., Zhang, Y., Jin, L., Luo, L., Xue, B., Lu, C., Zhang, X., Yin, Z.: Hsp70 inhibits lipopolysaccharide-induced NF-kappaB activation by interacting with TRAF6 and inhibiting its ubiquitination. FEBS Lett., 314: 1079-1086, 2006.

Fujimoto, S., Furue, H., Kimura, T., Kondo, T., Orita, K., Taguchi, T., Yoshida, K., Ogawa, N.: Clinical outcome of postoperative adjuvant immunochemotherapy with sizofiran for patients with resectable gastric cancer: a randomised controlled study. Eur. J. Cancer, 27: 1114–1118, 1991.

Hong, F., Hansen, R. D., Yan, J., Allendorf, D. J., Baran, J. T., Ostroff, G. R., Ross, G. D.: β-Glucan functions as an adjuvant for monoclonal antibody immunotherapy by recruiting tumoricidal granulocytes as killer cells. Cancer Res., 63: 9023-9031, 2003.

Hong, F., Yan, J., Baran, J. T., Allendorf, D. J., Hansen, R. D., Ostroff, G. R., Xing, P. X., Cheung, N. K., Ross, G. D.: Mechanism by which orally administered beta-glucans enhance the tumoricidal activity of antitumor monoclonal antibodies in murine tumor models. J. Immunol., 173: 797-806, 2004.

Itoh, W., Sugawara, I., Kimura, S., Tabata, K., Hirata, A., Kojima, T., Mori, S., Shimada, K.: Immunopharmacological study of sulfated schizophyllan (SPG). I. Its action as a mitogen and anti-HIV agent. Int. J. Immunopharmacol., 12: 225-233, 1990.

Kernodle, D. S., Gates, H., Kaiser, A. B.: Prophylactic anti-infective activity of poly-[1-6]-β-D-glucopyranosyl-[1-3]-β-D-glucopyranose glucan in guinea pig model of staphylococcal would infection. Antimicrobial Agents Chemotherap., 42: 545-549, 1998.

Kim, J. W., Cho, H. A. R., Ku, S. K.: Efficacy test of Polycan, a beta-glucan originated from *Aureobasidium pullulans* SM-2001, on anterior cruciate ligament transection and partial medial meniscectomy-induced-osteoarthritis rats. J. Microbiol. Biotechnol., 2012; 22: 274-282.

Nosalova, V., Bobek, P., Cerna, S., Galbavy, S., Stvrtina, S.: Effects of Pleuran (b-glucan isolated from *Pleurotus ostreatus*) on experimental colitis in rats. Physiol. Res., 50: 575-581, 2001.

Ostergren, K.: Reduced and high molecular weight barley beta-glucans decrease plasma total and non-HDL-cholesterol in hypercholesterolemic Syrian golden hamsters. J. Nutr., 134: 2617-2622, 2004.

Richter, J., Kral, V., Svozil, V., Rajnohova Dobiasova, L., Pohorska, J., Stiborova, I., Vetvicka, V.: Effects of Transfer Point Glucan #300 on children exposed to passive smoking – Placebo-driven double-blind clinical trials. J. Nutr. Health, 1:105-111, 2014 a

Richter, J., Svozil, V., Kral, V., Rajnohova Dobiasova, L., Stiborova, I., Vetvicka, V.: Clinical trials of yeast-derived β-(1,3) glucan in children: Effects on innate immunity. Ann. Trans. Med., 2, 2014 b. Doi:10.3978/j.issn.2305-5839.2014.02.01.

Richter, J., Svozil, V., Kral, V., Rajnohova Dobiasova, L., Stiborova, I., Vetvicka, V.: Clinical trials of yeast-derived β-(1,3) glucan in children: effects on innate immunity. Ann. Transl. Med., 2: 2, 2014 c. Doi:10.3978/j.issn.2305-5839.2014.02.01.

Senoglu, N., Yuzbasioglu, M. F., Aral, M., Ezberci, M., Kurutas, E. B., Bulbuloglu, E., Ezberci, F., Oksuz, H., Ciragil, P.: Protective effects on N-acetylcysteine and beta-glucan pretreatment on oxidative stress in cecal ligation and puncture model od sepsis. J. Invest. Surg., 21: 237-243, 2008.

Sima P, Vannucci L, Vetvicka V.: β-Glucans and cholesterol (Review). Int. J. Mol. Med., 41:1799-1808, 2018.

Tietyen J.L., Nevins D.J., Schneeman B.O., Characterization of the hypercholesterolemic potential of oat bran. FASEB J., *4: A527, 1990*.

Vannucci, L., Krizan, J., Sima, P., Stakheev, D., Caja, F., Raksiglova, L., Horak, V., Saieh, M.: Immunostimulatory properties and antitumor activities of glucan. Int. J. Oncol., 43: 357-364, 2013.

Vetvicka, V., Gover, O., Karpovsky, M., Hayby, H., Danay, O., Ezov, N., Hadar, Y., Schwartz, B.: Immune-modulating activities of glucans extracted from *Pleurotus ostreatus* and *Pleurotus eryngii*. J. Funct. Foods, 54: 81-91, 2019.

Vetvicka, V., Thornton, B. P., Wieman, T. J., Ross, G. D.: Targeting of NK cells to mammary carcinoma via naturally occurring tumor cell-bound iC3b and β-glucan-primed CR3 (CD11b/CD18). J. Immunol., 159: 599-605, 1997.

Vetvicka V., Vetvickova, J.: Physiological effects of different types of β-glucan. Biomed. Pap. Med. Fac. Univ. Palacky, 151: 225-231, 2007.

Vetvicka, V., Vetvickova, J.: Glucan supplementation enhances the immune response against an influenza challenge in mice. Ann. Transl. Med., 3, 2015, doi:10.3978/j.issn.2305-5839.2015.01.08.

Vetvicka, V., Vetvickova, J.: Comparison of immunological effects of commercially available β-glucans: Part III. Int. Clin. Pathol. J., 2, 2016, doi:10.15406/icpjl.2016.02.00046.

Wilson, T.A., Nicolosi, R.J., Delaney, B., Chadwell, K., Moolchandani, V., Kotyla, T., Ponduru, S., Zheng, G.H., Hess, R., Knutson, N., Curry, L., Kolberg, L., Goulson, M., Zhao, Q., Hu, X., Guo, Q., Gui, S.W., Xian, Y.: Physicochenical properties and regulatory effects in db/db diabetic mice of β-glucans extracted from oat, wheat and barley. Food Hydrocolloids, 37: 60-68, 2014.

16

COMPARISON

Nowadays, foods with health benefits have become very popular. Functional foods are regularly introduced into our diet. More and more manufacturers are jumping on the healthy food bandwagon, but not all extracts are created equal and their products differ widely in composition and, subsequently, in quality and activity. With very few comparative studies available, the consumer needs to do homework. Natural immunomodulators offering strong activity and no side effects have been sought for centuries. The current market is full of both individual immunomodulators and various combinations all promising the golden fleece-inexpensive and active stimulation of immune reactions.

Inexpensive and effective natural immunomodulators represent a holy grail of current alternative medicine. Some have been extensively studied for decades with an impressive number of peer-reviewed scientific papers (such as glucan), while some give confusing results based on isolation sources (such as *Echinacea*, where results widely differ based on the part of plant used for isolation) (Barret et al., 1999). When we consider some differences between individual batches, based on the natural source of material, it is understandable why big pharmaceutical companies still are not convinced. Some of the natural immunomodulators have already reached clinical trials and with dozens of clinical trials under way, their use in regular clinical practice is only a question of time. However, despite clear and well-established biological effects of this immunomodulator, the search for even better effects continues.

To date, very few papers have compared individual immunostimulators (Wilasrusmee et al., 2002, Saldanha and Tollefsbol, 2012). Based on the limited published comparisons, we decided to compare numerous commercially available immunostimulators. To do this, we used every immunomodulator mentioned in this book––*Astragalus*, ellagic acid, *Chlorella*, Cat's Claw, Glucan #300, ginseng, elderberry, thyme essential oil, and *Echinacea*––with only one aim, to test them against each other in well-established reactions. Discovering small natural molecules that regulate the immune system will increase our understanding of how diet and nutrition improve immune functions. The objective of this study was to compare individual natural molecules with demonstrated immunostimulating properties.

Stimulation of phagocytosis is usually the first effect of any natural immunomodulator. Using a model of synthetic polymeric 2-hydroxyethylmethacrylate microspheres, we measured the phagocytic activity after feeding with tested substances for two weeks. Our data are summarized in Figure 19 and show that only glucan and *Astragalus* significantly increased phagocytic activity of blood neutrophils and peritoneal macrophages

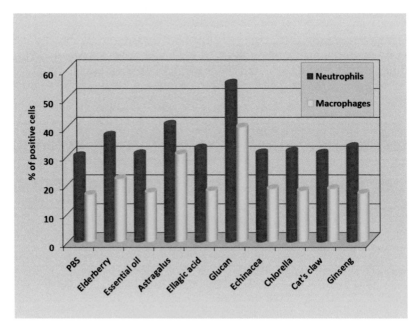

Figure 19 Effects on phagocytosis

The next part of our study focused on production of IL-2. IL-2 levels were measured after a 72-hr. *in vitro* incubation of spleen cells isolated from control and stimulant-treated animals. Since the secretion of IL-2 by nonstimulated cells (PBS) was always a zero, all tested material showed significant stimulation of IL-2 production (Figure 20). The most active materials were elderberry, *Astragalus*, ellagic acid, and glucan. Essential oil had no effects at all.

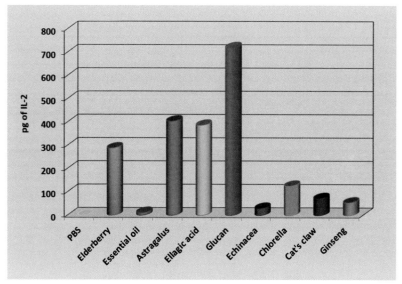

Figure 20 Effects on production of IL-2

Most natural immunomodulators stimulate cellular immunity; however, recent studies also showed significant effects on humoral branch. As an experimental model, we used immunization with ovalbumin as an antigen. Mice were injected twice with albumin and the serum was collected 7 days after the final injection. All tested samples stimulated antibody formation to some extent, with the glucan stimulation being by far the strongest (Figure 21).

Figure 21
Effects on antibody
formation

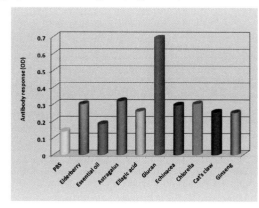

We then focused on the role of tested substances in cancer inhibition. Using a model of Lewis lung carcinoma cells, we showed that cyclophosphamide caused 70% inhibition of the number of lung metastases in comparison to the control group (Vetvicka et al., 2007). However, cyclophosphamide is a strong chemotherapeutic drug and we tried to find out if we can use a natural modulator instead. Our data summarized in Figure 22 show that only glucan significantly lowered the number of lung metastases. Whereas any of the tested materials showed only few percent inhibition (if any inhibition at all), glucan showing 47% inhibition

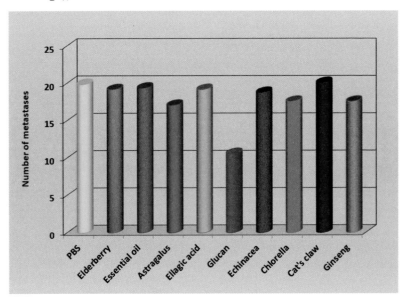

Figure 22 Effects on inhibition of lung cancer

Our last experiments focused on NK cell activity, which is an important immunological feature involved in numerous defense mechanisms, particularly in detection and elimination of viruses and cancer (Cerwenka and Lanier, 2016). Our experiments showed that some samples (e.g., essential oil) had no activity and others demonstrated mediocre activity (Figure 23).

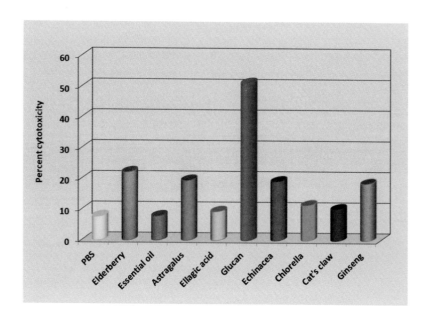

Figure 23 Effects on NK cell activity

The only supplement with high potential to activate NK cells was Glucan #300, which was already established both in animal (Vetvicka and Vetvickova, 2015) and human (Pohorska et al., 2016) models.

Several conclusions can be made—most of the commercial immunostimulating compounds have only very limited, if any, effects on the immune system including cancer. In addition, doses recommended on the label might not be sufficient, but no solid data on dosages exist with the exception of glucan (Vetvicka and Vetvickova, 2010). Experiments summarized in this Chapter clearly demonstrated that among all tested supplements, only glucan offered consistent immunoenhancing activities. Similar data were previously published (Vetvicka and Vetvickova, 2014). As glucan emerged as a clear winner, it is not surprising that direct comparisons of individual supplements do not exist, as most samples would be shown to have little or no activity. In this regards, individual commercial glucans were repeatedly tested against each other (Vetvicka and Vetvickova, 2005, 2007, 2010, 2014).

References

Barrett, B., Vohnmann, M., Calabrese, C.: *Echinacea* for upper respiratory infection. J. Fam. Practice, *48:* 628-635, 1999.

Cerwenka, A., Lanier, L.L.: Natural killer cell memory in infection, inflammation and cancer. Nature Rev. Immunol., 16:112-123, 2016.

Pohorska, J., Richter, J., Kral, V., Rajonohova Dobiasova, L., Stiborova, I., Vetvicka, V.: Reconstruction of NK cells during complex cancer treatment. J. Tumor, 4: 398-402, 2016.

Saldanha, S.N., Tollefsbol, T.O.: The role of nutraceuticals in chemoprevention and chemotherapy and their clinical outcomes. J. Oncol., 2012, doi:10.1155/2012/192464.

Vetvicka, V., Dvorak, B., Vetvickova, J., Richter, J., Krizan, J., Sima, P., Yvin, J-C: Orally-administered marine (1->3)-β-D-glucan Phycarine stimulates both humoral and cellular immunity. Int. J. Biol. Macromol., 40: 291-298, 2007.

Vetvicka, V., Vetvickova, J.: Immunostimulating properties of two different β-glucans isolated from maitake mushroom (*Grifola frondosa*). JANA 8: 33-39, 2005.

Vetvicka, V., Vetvickova, J.: Physiological effects of different types of beta-glucan. Biomed. Pap. Med. Fac. Univ. Palacky Olomouc Czech Repub., 151: 225-231, 2007.

Vetvicka, V., Vetvickova, J.: A comparison of injected and orally administered beta glucans. JANA 11: 42-49, 2008.

Vetvicka, V. Vetvickova, J.: b-1,3-glucan: Silver bullet of hot air? Open Glycoscience 3: 1-6, 2010.

Vetvicka, V., Vetvickova, J.: Natural immunomodulators and their stimulation of immune reaction: True or false? Anticancer Res., 34: 2275-2282, 2014.

Vetvicka, V., Vetvickova, J.: Glucan supplementation has strong anti-melanoma effects: Role of NK cells. Anticancer Res., 35: 5287-5292, 2015.

Wilasrusmee, C., Siddiqui, J., Brusch, D., Wilasrusmee, S., Kittur, S., Kittur, D.S.: *In vitro* immunomodulatory effects of herbal products. Am. Surg., 68: 860-854, 2002.

17

Conclusions

The importance of medicinal plants and individual extracts as complementary and alternative remedies is growing. Increasing quality and efficiency of novel drugs have not impacted the importance of natural products and the interest in these products.

Some people believe that old remedies are just better than synthetic products of the pharmaceutical industry, and some prefer cheaper natural products versus the expensive drugs with potential negative side effects. Not surprisingly, the marketing and consumer use of herbs and dietary supplements have risen dramatically in the USA over the past two decades (Timbo et al., 2006).

However, even natural products are not completely without problems. A main problem in characterizing natural products is identifying which of the numerous molecules found in the individual extract is responsible for the desired effects. In nature, they represent a complex mixture of ingredients, each of which might (and probably will) somehow contribute to biological activity.

Regardless of the country, there are dozens and most probably hundreds of different nutraceuticals available, strongly differing in quality, source, purity, and price. All proport the best effects under the sun. Which one should we buy? The most important aspect is to either manufacture or purchase any biological material from a solid source and control the quantity, purity, and the biological activity. Beware of middle-men and, if possible, buy directly from manufacturers or from resellers with clearly demonstrated connection to the manufacturers. We have to remember that one nutraceutical can be on the market under more than 10 commercial versions. When you do not know where it is manufactured, that might be the first red flag. In order to obtain the relevant information, it is imperative to get through the smoke and mirrors of unsupported or sometimes even pseudoscientific claims offered by the resellers. There are some telltale signs that should immediately raise another red flag. One of these is a full database of scientific papers without any direct proof that the research was done using the material the company is actually selling. It is very easy to find dozens of papers describing the biological effect of any nutraceutical, but if the particular study is not done for the material of interest, it is not relevant.

Our knowledge of biological and medicinal effects of the various medicinal plants and extracts is still beginning. Intensive but sometimes less focused research offers tantalizing possibilities, but any conclusions are still far from our reach. The wide range of herbal plants contains different chemical groups. We often know a lot about the direct effects of these individual phytochemicals, but much less about their effects when combined together. This could explain why it is so difficult to unequivocally recommend individual medicinal plants.

Another problem might be the potential increase of adverse events when herbs and dietary supplements are taken alone or concomitantly with medications. Many known problems are covered in the individual chapters. It is estimated that over 50% of patients with chronic diseases use some type of supplement. A majority of those patients never disclose that they are taking supplements to their healthcare providers. The five herbs/botanical products with the most interactions with individual medications were St. John's wort, ginkgo, kava, digitalis, and willow. Almost 20% of medications for nervous system conditions had negative interactions, followed by 17% for cardiovascular system, 15% for infection, and 12% for alimentary tract and metabolism. The three most sensitive drugs were warfarin, insulin, and digoxin. It is clear that patients using medications having a narrow therapeutic range were at greater risk of adverse reactions. It is important to note that this study did not find one reported negative side effects or interaction with glucan, making it the safest natural modulator on the market.

In summary, medical plants, herbs, and various natural molecules clearly have some, often positive, effect on our health. By no means are we trying to discourage the public from using natural immunomodulators. At the same time, it is imperative to note that not all immunomodulators are created equal. In many cases, we do not know enough about their actions, their actions and/or extract quality are dubious at best, or they have significant negative side effects. With the whole picture more in focus, glucan with biological effects backed by over 40,000 published scientific studies and no known negative side effects, is a clear winner.

References

Tsai, H.H., Lin, H.W., Pickard, A.S., Tsai, H.Y., Mahady, G.B.: Evaluation of documented drug interactions and contraindications associated with herbs and dietary supplements: a systematic literature review. Int. J. Clin. Pract., 66: 1056-1078, 2012.

Timbo, B.B., Ross, M.P., McCarthy, P.V., Lin, C.T.: Dietary supplements in a national survey: prevalence of use and reports of adverse events. J. Am. Diet. Assoc., 106: 1966-1974, 2006.